Emergency Department Operations and Administration

Editors

JOSHUA W. JOSEPH
BENJAMIN A. WHITE

EMERGENCY MEDICINE
CLINICS OF NORTH AMERICA

www.emed.theclinics.com

Consulting Editor
AMAL MATTU

August 2020 • Volume 38 • Number 3

ELSEVIER

1600 John F. Kennedy Boulevard • Suite 1800 • Philadelphia, Pennsylvania, 19103-2899

http://www.theclinics.com

EMERGENCY MEDICINE CLINICS OF NORTH AMERICA Volume 38, Number 3
August 2020 ISSN 0733-8627, ISBN-13: 978-0-323-73365-6

Editor: John Vassallo
Developmental Editor: Casey Potter

Emergency Medicine Clinics of North America (ISSN 0733-8627) is published quarterly by Elsevier Inc., 360 Park Avenue South, New York, NY, 10010-1710. Months of issue are February, May, August, and November. Business and Editorial Offices: 1600 John F. Kennedy Boulevard, Suite 1800, Philadelphia, PA 19103-2899. Customer Service Office: 6277 Sea Harbor Drive, Orlando, FL 32887-4800. Periodicals postage paid at New York, NY, and additional mailing offices. Subscription prices are $100.00 per year (US students), $352.00 per year (US individuals), $716.00 per year (US institutions), $220.00 per year (international students), $462.00 per year (international individuals), $882.00 per year (international institutions), $100.00 per year (Canadian students), $411.00 per year (Canadian individuals), and $882.00 per year (Canadian institutions). International air speed delivery is included in all *Clinics'* subscription prices. All prices are subject to change without notice. **POSTMASTER:** Send address changes to *Emergency Medicine Clinics of North America*, Elsevier Periodicals Customer Service, 11830 Westline Industrial Drive, St. Louis, MO 63146. Customer Service (orders, claims, online, change of address): Elsevier Periodicals **Customer Service, 11830 Westline Industrial Drive, St. Louis, MO 63146. Tel: 1-800-654-2452 (U.S. and Canada); 314-453-7041 (outside U.S. and Canada). Fax: 314-453-5170. E-mail: journalscustomerservice-usa@elsevier.com (for print support); journalsonlinesupport-usa@elsevier.com (for online support).**

Reprints. For copies of 100 or more of articles in this publication, please contact the Commercial Reprints Department, Elsevier Inc., 360 Park Avenue South, New York, NY 10010-1710. Tel.: 212-633-3874; Fax: 212-633-3820; E-mail: reprints@elsevier.com.

Emergency Medicine Clinics of North America is covered in *MEDLINE/PubMed (Index Medicus), Current Contents/Clinical Medicine, EMBASE/Excerpta Medica, BIOSIS, SciSearch, CINAHL, ISI/BIOMED,* and *Research Alert.*

Contributors

CONSULTING EDITOR

AMAL MATTU, MD
Professor and Vice Chair of Academic Affairs, Department of Emergency Medicine, University of Maryland School of Medicine, Baltimore, Maryland

EDITORS

JOSHUA W. JOSEPH, MD, MS, MBE
Director of Operations Research, Department of Emergency Medicine, Beth Israel Deaconess Medical Center, Assistant Professor of Emergency Medicine, Harvard Medical School, Boston, Massachusetts

BENJAMIN A. WHITE, MD
Director of Clinical Operations, Department of Emergency Medicine, Massachusetts General Hospital, Associate Professor of Emergency Medicine, Harvard Medical School, Boston, Massachusetts

AUTHORS

EMILY AARONSON, MD, MPH
Massachusetts General Hospital, Boston, Massachusetts

JARED S. ANDERSON, MD
The Warren Alpert Medical School, Brown University, Brown Emergency Medicine, Providence, Rhode Island

WILLIAM E. BAKER, MD
Associate Clinical Professor, Department of Emergency Medicine, Boston University, Boston University Medical Center, Boston, Massachusetts

CHRISTOPHER W. BAUGH, MD, MBA
Vice Chair of Clinical Affairs, Department of Emergency Medicine, Brigham and Women's Hospital, Boston, Massachusetts

LORNA M. BREEN, MD
Assistant Professor, Department of Emergency Medicine, Medical Director, Allen Hospital Emergency Department, Columbia University Vagelos College of Physicians and Surgeons, New York, New York

ALICE KIDDER BUKHMAN, MD, MPH
Director of Clinical Operations, Brigham and Women's Faulkner Emergency Department, Department of Emergency Medicine, Brigham and Women's Hospital, Boston, Massachusetts

BETTY C. CHANG, MD
Medical Director, Milstein Adult Emergency Department, NewYork-Presbyterian Hospital, Assistant Professor, Department of Emergency Medicine, Columbia University Irving Medical Center, New York, New York

ARLENE S. CHUNG, MD, MACM
Residency Director, Department of Emergency Medicine, Maimonides Medical Center, Brooklyn, New York

SAMUEL R. DAVIS, PhD
Northeastern University, Boston, Massachusetts

NICHOLAS GAVIN, MD, MBA, MS
Vice Chair of Clinical Operations, Assistant Professor, Department of Emergency Medicine, Columbia University Vagelos College of Physicians and Surgeons, New York, New York

KEITH C. HEMMERT, MD
Director of Operations, Hospital of University of Pennsylvania Emergency Department, Assistant Professor, Department of Emergency Medicine, Perelman School of Medicine, University of Pennsylvania, Philadelphia, Pennsylvania

NICOLE R. HODGSON, MD
Senior Associate Consultant, Department of Emergency Medicine, Mayo Clinic, Mayo Clinic Hospital, Phoenix, Arizona

DANA IM, MD, MPP, MPhil
Department of Emergency Medicine, Brigham and Women's Hospital, Boston, Massachusetts

BRYAN IMHOFF, MD, MBA
Assistant Professor, Department of Emergency Medicine, University of Kansas Medical Center, Kansas City, Kansas

JOSHUA W. JOSEPH, MD, MS, MBE
Director of Operations Research, Department of Emergency Medicine, Beth Israel Deaconess Medical Center, Assistant Professor of Emergency Medicine, Harvard Medical School, Boston, Massachusetts

JAMES F. KENNY, MD
Assistant Medical Director, Milstein Adult Emergency Department, NewYork-Presbyterian Hospital, Assistant Professor, Department of Emergency Medicine, Columbia University Irving Medical Center, New York, New York

EVAN L. LEVENTHAL, MD, PhD
Department of Emergency Medicine, Beth Israel Deaconess Medical Center, Harvard Medical School, Boston, Massachusetts

KENNETH D. MARSHALL, MD, MA
Associate Professor and Director of Clinical Operations, Associate Professor, Departments of Emergency Medicine, and History and Philosophy of Medicine, University of Kansas Medical Center, Kansas City, Kansas

LEON D. SANCHEZ, MD, MPH
Department of Emergency Medicine, Beth Israel Deaconess Medical Center, Boston, Massachusetts

KRAFTIN E. SCHREYER, MD
Department of Emergency Medicine, Temple University Hospital, Lewis Katz School of Medicine at Temple University, Philadelphia, Pennsylvania

JOSHUA J. SOLANO, MD
Assistant Professor of Emergency Medicine, Integrated Medical Science, Florida Atlantic University, Boca Raton, Florida

JONATHAN D. SONIS, MD, MHCM
Associate Director of Quality and Safety, Department of Emergency Medicine, Massachusetts General Hospital, Assistant Professor of Emergency Medicine, Harvard Medical School, Boston, Massachusetts

BRYAN A. STENSON, MD
Beth Israel Deaconess Medical Center, Harvard Medical School, Boston, Massachusetts

STEPHEN J. TRAUB, MD
Consultant and Chair, Department of Emergency Medicine, Mayo Clinic, Mayo Clinic Hospital, Phoenix, Arizona

RICHARD TREPP Jr. MD
Director of Informatics and Analytics, Assistant Professor, Department of Emergency Medicine, Columbia University Vagelos College of Physicians and Surgeons, New York, New York

DEBORAH VINTON, MD, MBA
Department of Emergency Medicine, University of Virginia Health System, Charlottesville, Virginia

BENJAMIN A. WHITE, MD
Director of Clinical Operations, Department of Emergency Medicine, Massachusetts General Hospital, Associate Professor of Emergency Medicine, Harvard Medical School, Boston, Massachusetts

MATTHEW L. WONG, MD, MPH
Assistant Professor, Department of Emergency Medicine, Beth Israel Deaconess Medical Center, Harvard Medical School, Boston, Massachusetts

BRIAN J. YUN, MD, MBA, MPH
Medical Director of ED Observation Unit, Department of Emergency Medicine, Massachusetts General Hospital, Boston, Massachusetts

FRANK ZILM, DArch, FAIA
Chester Dean Director of the Institute for Health + Wellness Design, University of Kansas School of Architecture, Lawrence, Kansas

Contents

Foreword: Emergency Department Operations and Administration   xiii

Amal Mattu

Preface: How the Emergency Department Works: A Work in Progress   xv

Joshua W. Joseph and Benjamin A. White

Emergency Department Operations: An Overview   549

Joshua W. Joseph and Benjamin A. White

Emergency department (ED) operations reflect the intersection of factors external and internal to the ED itself, with unique problems posed by community and academic environments. ED crowding is primarily caused by a lack of inpatient beds for patients admitted through the ED. Changes to front-end operations, such as point-of-care testing and putting physicians in triage, can yield benefits in throughput, but require individual cost analyses. Balancing physician workloads can lead to substantial improvements in throughput. Observation pathways can reduce crowding while maintaining safety. Physician and nurse well-being is an underappreciated topic within operations, and demands close attention and further research.

Queuing Theory and Modeling Emergency Department Resource Utilization   563

Joshua W. Joseph

Queueing theory is a discipline of applied mathematics that studies the behavior of lines. Queueing theory has successfully modeled throughput in a variety of industries, including within the emergency department (ED). Queueing equations model the demand for different processes within the ED, and help to factor in effects of variability on delays and service times. Utilization is a measure of the throughput of a process relative to demand, and provides a quick means of comparing the demand for certain resources. Although there have been some significant successes in applying queueing theory to EDs, the field remains underused within ED operations.

Factors Affecting Emergency Department Crowding   573

James F. Kenny, Betty C. Chang, and Keith C. Hemmert

Emergency department crowding is a multifactorial issue with causes intrinsic to the emergency department and to the health care system. Understanding that the causes of emergency department crowding span this continuum allows for a more accurate analysis of its effects and a more global consideration of potential solutions. Within the emergency department, boarding of inpatients is the most appreciable effect of hospital-wide crowding, and leads to further emergency department crowding. We explore the concept of emergency department crowding, and its causes, effects, and potential strategies to overcome this problem.

Staffing and Provider Productivity in the Emergency Department   589

Bryan A. Stenson, Jared S. Anderson, and Samuel R. Davis

Staffing and productivity are key concepts to understand when managing an emergency department. Provider productivity is not static, starts out high, and decreases throughout the shift in a stepwise manner. It is commonly measured by patients per hour or relative value units per hour, and is impacted by factors from the presence of residents to shift length. Appropriate staffing requires thorough understanding of the workforce and the variable patient demand of the department. Matching capacity to this demand potentially improves overall throughput and efficiency. Once knowledgeable about these factors, we provide a case study to showcase their application.

Patient Assignment Models in the Emergency Department   607

Nicole R. Hodgson and Stephen J. Traub

Early assignment of patients to specific treatment teams improves length of stay, rate of patients leaving without being seen, patient satisfaction, and resident education. Multiple variations of patient assignment systems exist, including provider-in-triage/team triage, fast-tracks/vertical pathways, and rotational patient assignment. The authors discuss the theory behind patient assignment systems and review potential benefits of specific models of patient assignment found in the current literature.

Design of the Academic Emergency Department   617

Kenneth D. Marshall, Bryan Imhoff, and Frank Zilm

This article introduces a clinical audience to the process of emergency department (ED) design, particularly relating to academic EDs. It explains some of the major terms, processes, and key decisions that clinical staff will experience as participants in the design process. Topics covered include an overview of the planning and design process, issues related to determining needed patient capacity, the impact of patient flow models on design, and a description of several common ED design types and their advantages and disadvantages.

Lean Process Improvement in the Emergency Department   633

Lorna M. Breen, Richard Trepp Jr., and Nicholas Gavin

Lean engineering is based on a process improvement strategy originally developed at Toyota and has been used in many different industries to maximize efficiency by minimizing waste. Lean improvement projects are frequently instituted in emergency departments in an effort to improve processes and thereby improve patient care. Such projects have been undertaken with success in many emergency departments in order to improve metrics such as door-to-provider time, left without being seen rate, and patient length of stay. By reducing waste in the system, Lean processes aim to maximize efficiency and minimize delay and redundancy to the extent possible.

Alternative Dispositions for Emergency Department Patients 647

Alice Kidder Bukhman, Christopher W. Baugh, and Brian J. Yun

Alternatives to inpatient admission have been shown to be safe and effective for a variety of clinical conditions and can help relieve emergency department (ED) and inpatient crowding. Evidence-based alternatives include use of rapid ED follow-up clinics, observation units, and home hospital programs. Use of accelerated diagnostic pathways and shared decision making can help support clinicians and patients in appropriately choosing an alternative disposition to traditional inpatient admission. However, many institutions struggle to fully embrace possible alternative depositions because of challenges of patient access, clinician and patient comfort with diagnostic uncertainty, and perceived medicolegal risks.

Quality Assurance in the Emergency Department 663

William E. Baker and Joshua J. Solano

Quality assurance (QA) of care in the emergency department encompasses activities ensuring that the care provided meets applicable standards. Health care delivery is complex and many factors affect quality of care. Thus, quantification of health care quality is challenging, especially with regard to attribution of outcomes to various factors contributing to such care. A critical component of the process of QA is determination of quality health care and the concept of (unjustified) deviation from the reference applicable standard of care.

Information Management in the Emergency Department 681

Evan L. Leventhal and Kraftin E. Schreyer

Information management in the emergency department (ED) is a challenge for all providers. The volume of information required to care for each patient and to keep the ED functioning is immense. It must be managed through varying means of communication and in connection with ED information systems. Management of information in the ED is imperfect; different modes and methods of identification, interpretation, action, and communication can be beneficial or harmful to providers, patients, and departmental flow. This article reviews the state of information management in the ED and proposes recommendations to improve the management of information in the future.

Best Practices in Patient Safety and Communication 693

Dana Im and Emily Aaronson

Emergency medicine is a high-risk area of medical practice, with a high rate of preventable adverse events. This is multifactorial, hinging on the myriad system and processes issues that complicate emergency care. Strong teamwork and communication have been identified as critical components for safe care in emergency medicine. Health care professionals and leaders within emergency medicine can implement solutions aimed at cultivating a strong safety culture, creating processes and system-based approaches to improve patient safety. This article provides an overview of the evidence-based approaches to improve patient safety and communication.

Optimizing Patient Experience in the Emergency Department   705

Jonathan D. Sonis and Benjamin A. White

Emergency department (ED) patient experience is a growing area of focus for leaders in the ED and throughout health care. While many factors intrinsic to the ED care environment add to the challenge of providing patients with an excellent experience, doing so holds many benefits, including improved patient compliance and health outcomes, improved workplace satisfaction and reduced provider and staff burnout, decreased malpractice risk, and increased revenue. Although wait time is a major driver of patient experience, provider and staff communication are critically important and excellent communication and perceived empathy may mitigate long waits, overcrowded environments, and other challenges.

Management of the Academic Emergency Department   715

Deborah Vinton and Leon D. Sanchez

Academic emergency departments (EDs) play a vital role in provision of emergency care and contribute to training of resident physicians. Academic EDs also generate innovations and discoveries through clinical research within academic medical centers. However, academic EDs face challenges when initiating operational process improvement efforts because of the medical complexity of patients, academic culture within academic medical centers, and variability in productivity and specialty training of trainees. To optimize operations within academic EDs, it is critical to understand characteristics shared by academic EDs, how to implement process improvement initiatives, trainee impact on ED operations, and how to promote operational research.

Strategies for Provider Well-Being in the Emergency Department   729

Matthew L. Wong and Arlene S. Chung

A variety of operational and administrative factors have the potential to decrease wellness and negatively impact emergency physicians, in terms of both their on-the-job performance and their long-term career satisfaction. Among these are the issues of workload balance, physiologic and circadian stresses, and larger issues of malpractice risk and institutional support. This overview covers both emerging research on how these problems affect emergency physicians and strategies to help mitigate these challenges.

EMERGENCY MEDICINE
CLINICS OF NORTH AMERICA

FORTHCOMING ISSUES

November 2020
Emergency Department Resuscitation
Michael E. Winters and Susan R. Wilcox,
Editors

February 2021
Neurologic Emergencies
Michael K. Abraham and Evie G.
Marcolini, *Editors*

May 2021
Emergencies in the Elderly Patient
Robert S. Anderson, Phillip D. Magidson,
and Danya Khoujah *Editors*

RECENT ISSUES

May 2020
Risk Management in Emergency Medicine
Lauren M. Nentwich, Jonathan S.
Olshaker, *Editors*

February 2020
Orthopedic Emergencies
Michael C. Bond and Arun Sayal, *Editors*

November 2019
Genitourinary Emergencies
Ryan Spangler and Joshua Moskovitz,
Editors

SERIES OF RELATED INTEREST

Orthopedic Clinics
https://www.orthopedic.theclinics.com/

THE CLINICS ARE NOW AVAILABLE ONLINE!
Access your subscription at:
www.theclinics.com

Foreword

Emergency Department Operations and Administration

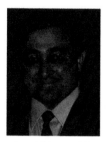

Amal Mattu, MD
Consulting Editor

Emergency Medicine Clinics of North America has always been one of the leading sources of cutting-edge information pertaining to the clinical practice of emergency medicine. The reader can frequently take what he or she has learned and apply it during the very next shift. So why in the world do we have an issue focused on emergency department (ED) operations and administration? To many readers, this doesn't sound very cutting edge or clinical, nor does it seem likely to be applicable to one's next shift.

Let me take you back 24 years…I recall in the spring of 1996 as I approached the end of my residency, our conference hosted a well-known guest speaker who was giving a talk on career choices. He asked my residency colleagues and me what we wanted to do with our careers. One of my fellow residents spoke up, "I want to find a place where I can just go to work, do my shifts, and then go home and not worry about anything else." The guest speaker, a veteran of emergency medicine for many years, responded, "That's a sure-fire way of burning out of this specialty." *Every other* senior member of the faculty nodded his or her head in agreement, and it left the rest of us junior doctors wondering why.

The guest speaker continued, "One of the biggest reasons burnout occurs in any specialty, especially in emergency medicine, is because physicians fail to take control of their work environment. They let other people or other circumstances dictate how they have to work…they feel powerless and victimized. If you want to have a successful and satisfying career in this specialty, you *have to* get involved. You *have to* learn how to control and improve the environment where you work." After more than 20 years of practice, I still remember that advice, and I've learned that it is absolutely true.

So why in the world does *Emergency Medicine Clinics of North America* have an issue focused on ED operations and administration? The reason is simple: we emergency physicians must take control of our working environment for the sake of our patients and for the sake of our own career satisfaction. Frontline emergency physicians

Emerg Med Clin N Am 38 (2020) xiii–xiv
https://doi.org/10.1016/j.emc.2020.05.004
0733-8627/20/© 2020 Published by Elsevier Inc.

are the very best people to make decisions about how their own EDs should function. For us to leave those decisions entirely up to hospital administrators who often know very little about the inner workings of an ED is truly a disservice to everyone who walks through the ED doors, patients and staff alike.

With those thoughts in mind, we present to you our first issue ever of *Emergency Medicine Clinics of North America* focused on ED operations and administration. This topic has been long overdue. Fortunately, guest editors Drs Josh Joseph and Ben White have stepped forward to present a fantastic issue discussing optimal approaches to various aspects of operations and administration. Basic issues that we face every day, such as ED overcrowding, patient dispositions, quality assurance, and information management, are addressed. They also take the reader a step deeper into operations with discussions on queuing theory and lean process improvement. An assortment of other administrative topics is addressed, including methods to optimize patient safety and the patient experience. They conclude with a discussion of provider well-being, acknowledging that patients are not the only participants whose satisfaction must always be addressed.

No emergency physician has the right to complain about their ED work environment unless he or she has made an attempt to improve it. The articles in this issue of *Emergency Medicine Clinics of North America* will carry you far in your journey of trying to improve your environment...for the sake of your patients and for the sake of yourself.

Amal Mattu, MD
Department of Emergency Medicine
University of Maryland School of Medicine
110 South Paca Street
6th Floor, Suite 200
Baltimore, MD 21201, USA

E-mail address:
amattu@som.umaryland.edu

Preface

How the Emergency Department Works: A Work in Progress

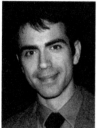 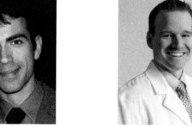

Joshua W. Joseph, MD, MS, MBE   Benjamin A. White, MD
Editors

Emergency medicine is a constantly changing field, and excellent emergency care requires clinicians to possess an intimate and broad knowledge of the principles of clinical care, and the principles needed to sustain a highly functioning emergency department (ED). To be an excellent emergency physician, empathy and a strong clinical acumen are prerequisites, but one must also understand the fundamentals of process flow, time management, team dynamics, efficient and effective communication, and quality improvement. The daily challenge of working in the ED is to actively manage these aspects of care while meeting many different patients' needs.

In this issue of *Emergency Medicine Clinics of North America*, we have attempted to provide a broad overview of current concepts relating to the growing field of ED operations. The authors have been asked to focus on blending the most current research in their fields with practical advice for emergency physicians. Not all of the information is necessarily something you can use on shift, although if you can rewrite troublesome features of your ED's information dashboard between seeing patients, more power to you, but many of the systems issues covered in these articles can and should be addressed by your physician staff as a group. And while many facets of operations research entail deep, technical analyses, sound emergency operations research always has the work of the frontline clinician and their patient's well-being as its ultimate concern.

The field of ED operations remains in constant flux, as the ED is often tasked with responding to larger issues in the health care system, and within society writ large. The issue of crowding has already challenged multiple generations of emergency physicians, reflecting broad gaps in availability for outpatient services, and the frequent misallocation of hospitals' inpatient capacity. For many EDs across North America, the only time there has been consistent respite from crowding has been in the middle of the COVID-19 pandemic, which has posed numerous operational challenges of its

Emerg Med Clin N Am 38 (2020) xv–xvi
https://doi.org/10.1016/j.emc.2020.05.003
0733-8627/20/© 2020 Published by Elsevier Inc.

emed.theclinics.com

own: from the need to coordinate the provision of protective equipment and ventilators to designing surge scheduling and novel workflows. Yet, this crisis, like many of the demand-capacity mismatches we have faced (and will continue to face) in emergency medicine, has further underscored the importance of understanding and leveraging the fundamental principles of ED operations.

Finally, we are lucky to have a contribution by the late Lorna M. Breen in this issue. Lorna was an active member of the emergency medicine operations community, a supportive colleague, and a dedicated clinician who cared deeply about her patients and the field of emergency medicine. We hope that future emergency physicians are inspired by her dedication to patient care, and to improving how the ED works, for those who are healed in it, and for those who do the hard, worthwhile work of healing in it.

Joshua W. Joseph, MD, MS, MBE
Department of Emergency Medicine
Beth Israel Deaconess Medical Center
Harvard Medical School
One Deaconess Road
Boston, MA 02215, USA

Benjamin A. White, MD
Department of Emergency Medicine
Massachusetts General Hospital
Harvard Medical School
MGH Emergency Medicine
Founders Building, Suite 852
Boston, MA 02114, USA

E-mail addresses:
jwjoseph@bidmc.harvard.edu (J.W. Joseph)
bwhite@mgh.harvard.edu (B.A. White)

Emergency Department Operations: An Overview

Joshua W. Joseph, MD, MS, MBE[a],*, Benjamin A. White, MD[b]

KEYWORDS

- Emergency department operations • Crowding • Throughput • Observation
- Efficiency

KEY POINTS

- Emergency department (ED) operations represent the systems and processes that are central to the provision of high-quality care in the ED.
- Emergency department operations reflect the intersection of clinical, economic, and cultural factors, and their effects on the care delivered in the emergency department.
- Although many of the factors affecting ED crowding are external to the emergency department, multiple options for considering process improvement along the spectrum of ED input, throughput, and output exist.
- In addition to improving patient flow, ED operational improvements can encompass a wide variety of themes including physical space design, process optimization, communication and patient experience, and staff wellness.

INTRODUCTION

"Why is this taking so long?" It is a question that patients often ask in the emergency department (ED), yet, it is also a question that emergency physicians often find themselves asking. Why is it that they are frequently working at capacity, walking up to several miles a shift,[1] all while neglecting to take any breaks to work faster, and everything is still taking so long to get done?

The answers lie within the domain of clinical operations, and more specifically the systems and processes designed to support provision of care in the ED. Although sometimes caused by the simple fact that a given system is poorly designed to meet its stated goal (eg, a demand-capacity mismatch in which resources are misallocated),[2] in many cases the interdependent processes needed to provide high-quality ED care require a more nuanced understanding of fundamental systems engineering principles, such as shifting bottlenecks, queuing theory, and so forth. In addition,

[a] Department of Emergency Medicine, Beth Israel Deaconess Medical Center, One Deaconess Road, Boston, MA 02215, USA; [b] Department of Emergency Medicine, Massachusetts General Hospital, 55 Fruit Street, Boston, MA 02114-2696, USA
* Corresponding author.
E-mail address: jwjoseph@bidmc.harvard.edu

Emerg Med Clin N Am 38 (2020) 549–562
https://doi.org/10.1016/j.emc.2020.04.005
0733-8627/20/© 2020 Elsevier Inc. All rights reserved.

emed.theclinics.com

although some systems inefficiencies and delays with inevitably always exist, there are myriad opportunities to optimize other patient care processes and patient experience, and these concepts are covered in detail elsewhere in this issue.

CROWDING AND THE MORAL IMPERATIVE OF EMERGENCY DEPARTMENT OPERATIONS MANAGEMENT

The need for careful operations management and further operations research in emergency medicine has never been more acute. For the past three decades, the most pressing barrier to effective ED operations has been the increasing degree of ED crowding, a phenomenon that is unfortunately present throughout the United States and internationally. The American College of Emergency Physicians' Emergency Medicine Practice Committee reports that more than 90% of EDs within the United States have reported frequently operating under crowded conditions.[3] Although the issue of crowding originally came under scrutiny during the late 1990s, there has yet to be a comprehensive solution implemented on a national, local, or regional level that meaningfully addresses the problem. In addition, ED crowding reflects the interaction of several distinct trends, which are active on a national scale, with issues that are unique to specific hospitals and EDs.[4,5]

The most significant systemic cause of crowding is that the demand for emergency care has continued to rise significantly relative to the availability of inpatient beds for admitted patients.[6,7] It is unclear what is driving the increase in ED visits, although potential causes proposed include the increased access to care provided by insurance coverage obtained under the auspices of the Affordable Care Act.[8,9] There has been a steady increase in certain disease burdens across the population, including drug and alcohol use disorders, and comorbidities of obesity,[10] which frequently lead to ED visits.

This has been paralleled by a substantial decrease in the proportion of low-acuity ED visits.[11] Much of this volume is thought to have been diverted to urgent-care clinics and similar facilities. Conversely, an increasing proportion of patients who require hospital admission are admitted directly through the ED, as a means of expediting laboratory testing, diagnostic imaging, and other workflows for the admission process.[12] The increasing acuity of ED visits may also reflect an increasing chronic disease burden concordant with the aging of the population.

Despite these trends of increasing ED use, there has been no concomitant increase in hospital inpatient capacity to meet the needs of patients requiring admission from the ED, and many hospitals have been reticent to implement improvements that have been shown to alleviate crowding.[5,13] Delays in admitting patients from the ED has been identified across numerous studies as a root cause of crowding.[6] Although hospitals' inpatient capacity and throughput is determined by a variety of social, cultural, regulatory, and economic factors, it is also likely that financial factors play a role, in that many hospitals generate more revenue from elective admissions than from ED admissions, especially given ED patients are more likely to be underinsured or uninsured.[14–16] As a result, many hospitals have little financial incentive to expand the proportion of their inpatient capacity available to patients admitted from the ED.

This represents a challenging moral problem, because the negative effects of crowding on patients, health care providers, and the health care system as a whole are legion. Crowding has been linked to significant decreases in the quality of care provided to patients, such as delayed time to the administration of antibiotics in pneumonia and in treatment of myocardial infarction, decreased compliance with core measures for sepsis, and decreased analgesia for patients with acute pain.[17–20]

Many of these deleterious effects may have an outsized impact on patients who are already suffering from significant health care disparities.[21] Crowding has been linked to increasing levels of burnout and moral distress among health care providers in the ED.[22–26] Finally, crowding has been linked to increases in the proportion of patients leaving the ED without being seen and rates of ambulance diversion.[27–29]

Common Challenges to Operations in Community Practice

In community practice, getting involved in operations is time-consuming and occasionally frustrating. The compensation afforded to ED medical directors varies significantly across institutions, as does the degree of agency that they may have relative to administrators, who might have neither direct clinical experience nor training in operations. Similarly, community physicians who volunteer their time to medical executive committees or focus groups, may find that doing so is difficult or impossible. Meetings may be scheduled without regard to shift-work and overnights. More consequentially, emergency physicians belonging to contract groups or corporate medical companies[30] may find themselves ineligible to sit on such committees, by dint of hospital policy. Most disturbingly, some corporate medicine practices have retaliated against physicians who have reported concerns about the quality of care and issues with ED administration.[30,31]

Challenges to Progress in Emergency Department Operations Research

Operations research within emergency medicine faces unique hurdles. Many traditional paradigms for clinical research cannot be translated into the operational domain. Although a physician and patient can both be blinded to which medication is administered during a randomized control trial, an emergency physician cannot be blinded to a change in the length of the shift she works, nor to whether she assigns herself patients or receives those assignments from a nurse manager. Even less robust trial designs, such as alternating day paradigms, are problematic to implement. A study examining changes to a single area of the ED, such as triage, might necessitate major changes to downstream workflows, making it difficult to change over a short interval. As a result, many operational research studies are only feasible as quasi-experimental (before-and-after) studies of planned changes to workflows.

The significance of results and end points of operations research often have little correspondence to those of outcomes measured within clinical and public health research. A 1% change in the sensitivity or specificity of a diagnostic test rarely provides a meaningful impetus to change practices. However, an improvement of similar magnitude in an ED's average length of stay could mean the difference between a safety-net ED's ongoing viability and closure. Differences in workflows used by different EDs also make multicenter studies hard to conduct and to interpret. Adding scribes to two EDs with similar volumes, physician staff sizes, and patient populations, but with different electronic medical record systems, could yield significant but completely contradictory outcomes at both sites.

CURRENT TRENDS IN EMERGENCY DEPARTMENT OPERATIONS RESEARCH

The root causes of ED crowding demand systemic redress, and are likely to remain in place for the foreseeable future. However, there exist major areas where improvements in efficiency and throughput can have a significant impact on crowding and the quality of patient care, despite the challenges of output factors described previously (**Fig. 1**). Many of the most exciting recent developments within the ED operations literature reflect attempts to make the best of the resources available to the ED,

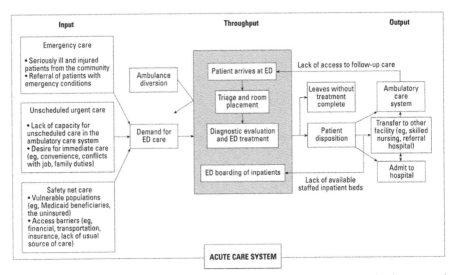

Fig. 1. Asplin input-throughput-output model. (*From* Asplin BR, Magid DJ, Rhodes KV, et al. A conceptual model of emergency department crowding. *Ann Emerg Med.* 2003 Aug;42(2):173-80; with permission.)

including strategies to more efficiently align existing diagnostic testing resources with demand, measures to better quantify throughput and optimize physician productivity, and alternative pathways to prevent inpatient admissions and acute hospital transfers. Although many of these themes are described elsewhere in this issue, a few interventions are worthy of discussion here.

INNOVATIONS TO DIAGNOSTIC TESTING AND RESOURCE ALLOCATION
Point-of-Care Testing

Point-of-care tests have long been an appealing alternative to traditional laboratory diagnostic tests thanks to their rapid turnaround time, but their accuracy and cost-effectiveness have been disputed.[32,33] Over the last decade, studies have demonstrated that point-of-care tests used in the ED setting can provide rapid results at slightly greater costs than traditional laboratory assays, but with comparable accuracy.[32,34] Although concerns about the tests' accuracy have somewhat abated, their limited cost-effectiveness is likely caused by the fact that laboratory testing is only a rate-limiting step for select patients. The most robust evidence demonstrating increased throughput with point-of-care testing addresses specific diagnostic scenarios, such as in obtaining creatinine to determine kidney function before contrast-enhanced computed tomography scans.[35–38] A similarly promising venue is for conditions in which care is protocolized, and in which laboratory testing significantly impacts a patient's disposition, such as in serial troponin measurements for chest pain.[39]

Nursing Protocols

Nursing triage protocols using standardized order sets for diagnostic tests and certain therapeutic interventions have been shown to improve throughput and improve quality measures, such as time-to-analgesia.[40] The best evidence for an effect of nursing protocols on improving patient throughput comes from protocols that are based on established evidence-based decision rules (eg, the Ottawa Ankle Rule), although some studies have suggested that by reducing time-to-analgesia, patient throughput is improved as a result.[41,42] Although the overall evidence for nursing protocols improving overall patient throughput remains limited because of the small sample sizes and methodological limitations of prior studies, the potential harms and costs associated with nurse-initiated treatments, such as nonnarcotic analgesia and β-agonists in pediatric asthma, are low and the potential benefits are considerable.[43]

Alternative Triage Workflows

Studies examining use of an emergency physician at triage have shown several improvements across a broad variety of operational metrics, including patient throughput.[38,44–46] A significant part of this effect on throughput may come from the accelerated ordering of diagnostic testing provided by the physician triage evaluation process.[38] Several of the quality benchmarks that the physician-triage process improves are endogenous variables: if a physician sees patients shortly after their arrival in the waiting room, then such measures as the door-to-doctor time and the rate of patients leaving without being seen improve irrespective of any change in overall throughput. Although a growing body of literature suggests that physician triage can improve patient throughput, its cost-effectiveness is not widely reported, and evidence suggests that it is most effective when performed by attending physicians, rather than midlevel practitioners or resident physicians.[47] Until more robust cost-effectiveness data are available, EDs should consider physician triage on a case-by-case basis, particularly when waiting room volumes are disproportionately high relative to other areas within the ED.

One potential offshoot of physician triage that has generated considerable interest is telemedicine physician triage. Telemedicine physician triage has the advantage of flexibility and potentially lower costs, because physicians may staff it remotely and can be activated at times of increased demand and prolonged wait times. Although only a few studies have been conducted examining it to date, they have generally demonstrated equivalent rates of safety and patient satisfaction, suggesting that this may be a viable alternative.[48–50]

THROUGHPUT, PRODUCTIVITY, PHYSICIAN SCHEDULING, AND WORKFLOW ADVANCEMENTS
Measuring Throughput and Productivity

Efforts to evaluate patient throughput as a function of physician productivity, and to further understand the dynamics of the productivity of individual emergency physicians have expanded considerably in recent years. Although previous paradigms of emergency physician productivity had examined productivity as a static average calculated over a shift,[51,52] more recent work suggests that when emergency physicians are responsible for seeing patients at their own pace, productivity tends to begin at a peak pace, and slowly declines over successive hours of a shift.[53,54] This progressive decrease in productivity has several mutually compatible explanations, including the mechanistic challenge of managing a growing roster of patients; decision fatigue; and so-called social loafing, the tendency to decrease work when relief is in sight.[55,56] However, current discussions of physician productivity remain limited in part by the lack of an agreed-on metric of work.

The most natural measure of throughput and physician productivity is the number of patients a physician sees per hour. This has a face validity, because patients are the ones to whom emergency care is provided, and throughput and crowding are fundamentally measured by the number of patients in the ED and waiting room at a given time. However, this measure belies that the amount of work to take care of patients varies drastically. Although combining this number with patient-level measures of acuity (eg, Emergency Severity Index) is an appealing compromise, doing so elides that acuity and effort are not directly related. For instance, a patient with a higher Emergency Severity Index level, but with care that is highly protocolized, such as a patient with an ST-segment elevation myocardial infarction, may take considerably less time to treat and disposition than a patient with abdominal pain who has a complex medical history.

Relative value units (RVUs) are an alternative measure of productivity tied to compensation, which have the appealing benefit of factoring in elements of the complexity of a history and physical, and measuring procedures. Given their close ties to compensation, they are an essential measure for cost-benefit measurements and projections. However, RVUs are a problematic measure for productivity relative to patient throughput and as a sole measure of physician workload. As in the case of patients per hour, RVUs do not necessarily correlate to the amount of work required to care for a given patient, and are heavily skewed toward procedures. The RVUs provided for a given patient encounter are also directly dependent on a physician's documentation, so two physicians seeing the same patients or performing the same procedures can generate substantially different numbers of RVUs.[57] Finally, the number of RVUs assigned to a procedure may vary significantly from year to year, making comparisons unreliable across time.

Novel Approaches to Physician Workflow and Shifts

Redesigning physician shift schedules and workflows to better align with patient volumes has shown significant potential to improve throughput and enhance patient safety. Approaches to optimizing physician shift schedules have ranged from those using tools that are complex, such as queueing theory and discrete event simulation models, to more straightforward approaches, such as roughly aligning physician schedules with times of higher patient arrivals.[58–61] Many of these studies have suggested that marked improvements in throughput and left without being seen rates are achieved through small realignments of physician schedules. However, with the noted exception of the landmark study by Green and colleagues[58] on the use of a queueing analysis to optimize a community hospital's shift schedule, there have been many simulated analyses of emergency physician staffing and few reports of real-world implementation, suggesting that this varied toolset has yet to be widely embraced.[62]

One of the most promising workflow designs entering use is rotational patient assignment. Originally described in the context of nurse-physician teams, rotational patient assignment consists of assigning patients alternatively to teams of clinicians as they arrive, rather than allowing physicians to assign themselves to patients at their own pace.[63,64] Rotational assignment is a distinct alternative to ED zones, which establish separate patient queues based on geography. Rotational assignment enforces a discipline of steady workflow, eliminating the unconscious tendency of emergency physicians to "peak" early in their shift, which is associated with decreased overall productivity,[65] and reduces spikes in arrivals across multiple teams, leading to robust decreases in door-to-doctor times, left without being seen rates, and overall patient length of stay.[66,67] Modern implementations of rotational patient assignment use a computer algorithm to distribute arrivals between teams, suggesting that machine learning approaches may have a future role in load-balancing teams over the course of shifts.

ALTERNATIVE SYSTEMS OF PATIENT ARRIVALS AND DISPOSITION
Observation Care and Observation Pathways

A lack of inpatient beds for admitted patients is a major driver of ED crowding, whereas conversely, strategies to reduce hospital admissions through ED-based observation units have demonstrated admirable cost-effectiveness relative to inpatient care.[68–72] Placing patients in ED observation care directly decreases the demand for inpatient beds, and a robust body of evidence demonstrates that for many conditions, such as low-risk chest pain, syncope, new-onset atrial fibrillation, and cellulitis, 24-hour observation within the ED following protocolized guidelines can substantially decrease patients' overall length of stay without an appreciable incidence of adverse outcomes.[69,73,74] The population of inpatients eligible for ED observation care represents a much wider variety of conditions beyond those that have common observation pathways.[75] Many of the patients who are cared for within observation units may leave the hospital considerably faster than they might otherwise if they were admitted to an inpatient ward or still boarding within the ED, and this likely represents the salutatory effects on crowding that have been observed in hospitals that have implemented ED observation units.[76] Many hospitals are also considering other alternatives to admission models of care, including home hospital and mobile observation unit models; however, further studies of effectiveness and scalability are needed.

Managing Patient Inflow and Secondary Disposition

A complementary set of strategies used by some EDs is to actively manage patient inflow and outflow. Several centers have described successfully directing lower-acuity patients (many of whom might otherwise go into a traditional fast-track setting) into designated "vertical care" areas. These areas consist of groups of chairs or recliners that can serve as intermediate waiting areas (when patients are taken to a separate area for examination and testing) or as a comprehensive space for patient care. Incorporating vertical areas has been shown to significantly improve throughput for lower-acuity complaints.[77–79]

A related intervention is transferring patients who are identified as falling within certain low-risk parameters directly to primary care or urgent care clinic appointments. Although this has not been widely adopted, it may be appealing to EDs with close relationships to affiliated primary or urgent care clinics.[80] Alternative strategies for diverting lower-acuity patients have been trialed across a variety of settings (including prehospital), but the results of these studies have been anecdotal and conflicting.[81] For hospitals with nearby affiliate sites, secondary disposition, in which a patient is treated in one ED, but transferred within network to another site with available inpatient beds, is a useful option to actively minimize boarding and crowding whenever inpatient beds are in short supply.[82]

Some hospitals have seen improvements with the implementation of a hospital-wide "full-capacity protocol." Full-capacity protocols leverage changes across hospital inpatient wards, such as expediting discharges and moving ED boarders to inpatient hallway beds. Although these protocols are an effective means of reducing crowding specifically at times of high admission volumes, their effectiveness may depend significantly on how consistently hospitals implement the protocol, and on the degree of cooperation from inpatient stakeholders. A designated hospital "bed czar" or nurse navigator can help to facilitate compliance with these protocols, and can smooth inpatient flow during less critical periods.[83,84]

FUTURE DIRECTIONS OF EMERGENCY DEPARTMENT OPERATIONS RESEARCH AND DEVELOPMENT
Measures Examining Physician Practice Patterns

The rates at which emergency physicians order diagnostic imaging and admit patients can have an outsized effect on overall throughput in the ED.[85] There is considerable variation in emergency physicians' practice patterns for ordering imaging, even when there are well-known evidence-based guidelines for practice, such as for computed tomography imaging in patients with low-risk head injury.[86,87] An emerging body of evidence implies that more conservative (and resource-intensive) practice patterns are correlated.[88] Although embedding decision support for imaging within electronic medical records is an appealing way to combat overuse, studies of its effectiveness have shown mixed results, potentially reflecting a host of causes for overuse.[89–91] More research is needed to understand the causes of these variations and to address them, but they represent some of the greatest areas for improvement within the ED itself.

Strategies to Optimize Physician Well-Being

Physician well-being, resilience, and burnout likely exert significant effects on the quality and efficiency of care delivered within the ED, and may help to explain some of the practice variation among emergency physicians.[92] Recent research suggests that the degree of burnout reported by emergency physicians' can serve as a predictor of the waiting times that their patients will experience as they go on shift, independent of other factors including the time of day and department census.[93] Emergency physicians report giving suboptimal care as their sense of burnout increases, and burnout among physicians has been broadly linked to higher rates of errors.[94,95]

Although enthusiasm for investigating burnout and resilience is growing, tangible solutions remain elusive.[96] Future avenues for improving physicians' resilience include investigating the roles of shift timing, length, and sleep patterns on cognitive performance and physiologic measures of stress.[97,98] Efforts to reduce the degree of overhead and interruptions emergency physicians face from electronic health records and alerts have the potential to reduce burnout and directly improve physicians' on-shift efficiency.[99,100]

SUMMARY

ED operations management poses challenges to physicians and researchers, stemming from factors external to the ED. Although these challenges are substantial, ED medical directors and even individual emergency physicians can still make important changes that can improve throughput and patient care. Emergency physicians have a duty to advocate for the resources needed to provide quality care for their patients, but also to help ensure that the work of emergency medicine does not require them to run themselves ragged in the process.

DISCLOSURE

The authors have nothing to disclose.

REFERENCES

1. Peters GA, Wong ML, Sanchez LD. Pedometer-measured physical activity among emergency physicians during shifts. Am J Emerg Med 2019;38(1):118–21. Available

at: http://www.sciencedirect.com/science/article/pii/S0735675719304668. Accessed November 4, 2019.

2. Rogg JG, Huckman R, Lev M, et al. Describing wait time bottlenecks for ED patients undergoing head CT. Am J Emerg Med 2017;35(10):1510–3.

3. American College of Emergency Physicians: Emergency Medicine Practice Committee. Emergency department crowding: high impact solutions. 2016. Available at: https://www.acep.org/globalassets/sites/acep/media/crowding/empc_crowding-ip_092016.pdf. Accessed October 1, 2019.

4. Morley C, Unwin M, Peterson GM, et al. Emergency department crowding: a systematic review of causes, consequences and solutions. PLoS One 2018; 13(8):e0203316. Available at: https://www.ncbi.nlm.nih.gov/pmc/articles/PMC6117060/. Accessed November 4, 2019.

5. Chang AM, Cohen DJ, Lin A, et al. Hospital strategies for reducing emergency department crowding: a mixed-methods study. Ann Emerg Med 2018;71(4): 497–505.e4.

6. Hoot NR, Aronsky D. Systematic review of emergency department crowding: causes, effects, and solutions. Ann Emerg Med 2008;52(2):126–36.e1.

7. Sun R, Karaca Z, Wong H. Trends in hospital emergency department visits by age and payer, 2006-2015 HCUP statistical brief #238. Rockville, MD: Agency for Healthcare Research and Quality; 2018. Available at: https://www.hcup-us.ahrq.gov/reports/statbriefs/sb238-Emergency-Department-Age-Payer-2006-2015.pdf. Accessed November 4, 2019.

8. Nikpay S, Freedman S, Levy H, et al. Effect of the Affordable Care Act Medicaid expansion on emergency department visits: evidence from state-level emergency department databases. Ann Emerg Med 2017;70(2):215–25.e6.

9. Dresden SM, Powell ES, Kang R, et al. Increased emergency department use in Illinois after implementation of the patient protection and affordable care act. Ann Emerg Med 2017;69(2):172–80.

10. Mokdad AH, Ballestros K, Echko M, et al. The state of US health, 1990-2016: burden of diseases, injuries, and risk factors among US states. JAMA 2018; 319(14):1444–72.

11. Poon SJ, Schuur JD, Mehrotra A. Trends in visits to acute care venues for treatment of low-acuity conditions in the United States from 2008 to 2015. JAMA Intern Med 2018 01;178(10):1342–9.

12. Schuur JD, Venkatesh AK. The growing role of emergency departments in hospital admissions. N Engl J Med 2012;367(5):391–3.

13. Warner LSH, Pines JM, Chambers JG, et al. The most crowded US hospital emergency departments did not adopt effective interventions to improve flow, 2007-10. Health Aff (Millwood) 2015;34(12):2151–2159A.

14. McHugh M, Regenstein M, Siegel B. The profitability of medicare admissions based on source of admission. Acad Emerg Med 2008;15(10):900–7.

15. Schuur JD. Overcrowded emergency departments: is sunlight enough of a disinfectant? JAMA Intern Med 2014;174(11):1846–7.

16. Moskop JC, Sklar DP, Geiderman JM, et al. Emergency department crowding. Part 1: concept, causes, and moral consequences. Ann Emerg Med 2009; 53(5):605–11.

17. Pines JM, Hollander JE, Localio AR, et al. The association between emergency department crowding and hospital performance on antibiotic timing for pneumonia and percutaneous intervention for myocardial infarction. Acad Emerg Med 2006;13(8):873–8.

18. Fee C, Weber EJ, Maak CA, et al. Effect of emergency department crowding on time to antibiotics in patients admitted with community-acquired pneumonia. Ann Emerg Med 2007;50(5):501–9.e1.

19. Pines JM, Hollander JE. Emergency department crowding is associated with poor care for patients with severe pain. Ann Emerg Med 2008;51(1):1–5.

20. Shin TG, Jo IJ, Choi DJ, et al. The adverse effect of emergency department crowding on compliance with the resuscitation bundle in the management of severe sepsis and septic shock. Crit Care 2013;17(5):R224.

21. Pines JM, Localio AR, Hollander JE. Racial disparities in emergency department length of stay for admitted patients in the United States. Acad Emerg Med 2009; 16(5):403–10.

22. Fernandez-Parsons R, Rodriguez L, Goyal D. Moral distress in emergency nurses. J Emerg Nurs 2013;39(6):547–52.

23. Popa F, Arafat R, Purcărea V, et al. Occupational burnout levels in emergency medicine: a nationwide study and analysis. J Med Life 2010;3(3):207–15.

24. Wolf LA, Perhats C, Delao AM, et al. "It's a burden you carry": describing moral distress in emergency nursing. J Emerg Nurs 2016;42(1):37–46.

25. Moskop JC, Geiderman JM, Marshall KD, et al. Another look at the persistent moral problem of emergency department crowding. Ann Emerg Med 2019; 74(3):357–64.

26. Chang BP, Cato KD, Cassai M, et al. Clinician burnout and its association with team based care in the emergency department. Am J Emerg Med 2019; 37(11):2113–4. Available at: http://www.sciencedirect.com/science/article/pii/S0735675719304139. Accessed November 4, 2019.

27. Weiss SJ, Ernst AA, Derlet R, et al. Relationship between the National ED Overcrowding Scale and the number of patients who leave without being seen in an academic ED. Am J Emerg Med 2005;23(3):288–94.

28. Kulstad EB, Hart KM, Waghchoure S. Occupancy rates and emergency department work index scores correlate with leaving without being seen. West J Emerg Med 2010;11(4):324–8.

29. Carter EJ, Pouch SM, Larson EL. The relationship between emergency department crowding and patient outcomes: a systematic review. J Nurs Scholarsh 2014;46(2):106–15.

30. Derlet RW, McNamara RM, Plantz SH, et al. Corporate and hospital profiteering in emergency medicine: problems of the past, present, and future. J Emerg Med 2016;50(6):902–9.

31. McNamara RM, Beier K, Blumstein H, et al. A survey of emergency physicians regarding due process, financial pressures, and the ability to advocate for patients. J Emerg Med 2013;45(1):111–6.e3.

32. Asha SE, Chan ACF, Walter E, et al. Impact from point-of-care devices on emergency department patient processing times compared with central laboratory testing of blood samples: a randomised controlled trial and cost-effectiveness analysis. Emerg Med J 2014;31(9):714–9.

33. Somma SD, Zampini G, Vetrone F, et al. Opinion paper on utility of point-of-care biomarkers in the emergency department pathways decision making. Clin Chem Lab Med 2014;52(10):1401–7.

34. McIntosh BW, Vasek J, Taylor M, et al. Accuracy of bedside point of care testing in critical emergency department patients. Am J Emerg Med 2018;36(4): 567–70.

35. Lee-Lewandrowski E, Chang C, Gregory K, et al. Evaluation of rapid point-of-care creatinine testing in the radiology service of a large academic medical

center: impact on clinical operations and patient disposition. Clin Chim Acta 2012;413(1):88–92.

36. You JS, Chung YE, Park JW, et al. The usefulness of rapid point-of-care creatinine testing for the prevention of contrast-induced nephropathy in the emergency department. Emerg Med J 2013;30(7):555–8.

37. Singer AJ, Williams J, Taylor M, et al. Comprehensive bedside point of care testing in critical ED patients: a before and after study. Am J Emerg Med 2015;33(6):776–80.

38. Singer AJ, Taylor M, LeBlanc D, et al. Early point-of-care testing at triage reduces care time in stable adult emergency department patients. J Emerg Med 2018;55(2):172–8.

39. Slagman A, von Recum J, Möckel M, et al. Diagnostic performance of a high-sensitive troponin T assay and a troponin T point of care assay in the clinical routine of an emergency department: a clinical cohort study. Int J Cardiol 2017;230:454–60.

40. Douma MJ, Drake CA, O'Dochartaigh D, et al. A pragmatic randomized evaluation of a nurse-initiated protocol to improve timeliness of care in an urban emergency department. Ann Emerg Med 2016;68(5):546–52.

41. Rowe BH, Villa-Roel C, Guo X, et al. The role of triage nurse ordering on mitigating overcrowding in emergency departments: a systematic review. Acad Emerg Med 2011;18(12):1349–57.

42. Hughes JA, Brown NJ, Chiu J, et al. The relationship between time to analgesic administration and emergency department length of stay: a retrospective review. J Adv Nurs 2020;76(1):183–90. Available at: http://onlinelibrary.wiley.com/doi/abs/10.1111/jan.14216. Accessed November 2, 2019.

43. Cabilan CJ, Boyde M. A systematic review of the impact of nurse-initiated medications in the emergency department. Australas Emerg Nurs J 2017;20(2):53–62.

44. Imperato J, Morris DS, Binder D, et al. Physician in triage improves emergency department patient throughput. Intern Emerg Med 2012;7(5):457–62.

45. Cheng I, Lee J, Mittmann N, et al. Implementing wait-time reductions under Ontario government benchmarks (pay-for-results): a cluster randomized trial of the effect of a physician-nurse supplementary triage assistance team (MDRNSTAT) on emergency department patient wait times. BMC Emerg Med 2013;13(1):17.

46. Rogg JG, White BA, Biddinger PD, et al. A long-term analysis of physician triage screening in the emergency department. Acad Emerg Med 2013;20(4):374–80.

47. Abdulwahid MA, Booth A, Kuczawski M, et al. The impact of senior doctor assessment at triage on emergency department performance measures: systematic review and meta-analysis of comparative studies. Emerg Med J 2016;33(7):504–13.

48. Tolia V, Castillo E, Guss D. EDTITRATE (Emergency Department Telemedicine Initiative to Rapidly Accommodate in Times of Emergency). J Telemed Telecare 2017;23(4):484–8.

49. Izzo JA, Watson J, Bhat R, et al. Diagnostic accuracy of a rapid telemedicine encounter in the emergency department. Am J Emerg Med 2018;36(11):2061–3.

50. Rademacher NJ, Cole G, Psoter KJ, et al. Use of telemedicine to screen patients in the emergency department: matched cohort study evaluating efficiency and patient safety of telemedicine. JMIR Med Inform 2019;7(2):e11233.

51. Arya R, Salovich DM, Ohman-Strickland P, et al. Impact of scribes on performance indicators in the emergency department. Acad Emerg Med 2010; 17(5):490–4.

52. Hamden K, Jeanmonod D, Gualtieri D, et al. Comparison of resident and midlevel provider productivity in a high-acuity emergency department setting. Emerg Med J 2014;31(3):216–9.

53. Joseph JW, Henning DJ, Strouse CS, et al. Modeling hourly resident productivity in the emergency department. Ann Emerg Med 2017;70(2):185–90.e6.

54. Joseph JW, Davis S, Wilker EH, et al. Modelling attending physician productivity in the emergency department: a multicentre study. Emerg Med J 2018;35(5): 317–22.

55. Laxmisan A, Hakimzada F, Sayan OR, et al. The multitasking clinician: decision-making and cognitive demand during and after team handoffs in emergency care. Int J Med Inf 2007;76(11):801–11.

56. Song H, Tucker AL, Murrell KL. The diseconomies of queue pooling: an empirical investigation of emergency department length of stay. Manag Sci 2015; 61(12):3032–53.

57. Martin DR, Moskop JC, Bookman K, et al. Compensation models in emergency medicine: an ethical perspective. Am J Emerg Med 2020;38(1):138–42. Available at: http://www.sciencedirect.com/science/article/pii/S0735675719305029. Accessed November 4, 2019.

58. Green LV, Soares J, Giglio JF, et al. Using queueing theory to increase the effectiveness of emergency department provider staffing. Acad Emerg Med 2006; 13(1):61–8.

59. Wang T, Guinet A, Belaidi A, et al. Modelling and simulation of emergency services with ARIS and Arena. Case study: the emergency department of Saint Joseph and Saint Luc Hospital. Production Planning & Control 2009;20(6):484–95.

60. Hung GR, Whitehouse SR, O'Neill C, et al. Computer modeling of patient flow in a pediatric emergency department using discrete event simulation. Pediatr Emerg Care 2007;23(1):5–10.

61. Wutthisirisart P, Martinez G, Heaton HA, et al. Maximizing patient coverage through optimal allocation of residents and scribes to shifts in an emergency department. J Med Syst 2018;42(11):212.

62. Saghafian S, Austin G, Traub SJ. Operations research/management contributions to emergency department patient flow optimization: review and research prospects. IIE Trans Healthc Syst Eng 2015;5(2):101–23.

63. DeBehnke D, Decker MC. The effects of a physician-nurse patient care team on patient satisfaction in an academic. Am J Emerg Med 2002;20(4):267–70.

64. Patel PB, Vinson DR. Team assignment system: expediting emergency department care. Ann Emerg Med 2005;46(6):499–506.

65. Joseph JW, Novack V, Wong ML, et al. Do slow and steady residents win the race? Modeling the effects of peak and overall resident productivity in the emergency department. J Emerg Med 2017;53(2):252–9.

66. Traub SJ, Bartley AC, Smith VD, et al. Physician in triage versus rotational patient assignment. J Emerg Med 2016;50(5):784–90.

67. Traub SJ, Saghafian S, Bartley AC, et al. The durability of operational improvements with rotational patient assignment. Am J Emerg Med 2018;36(8):1367–71.

68. Goodacre SW, Morris FM, Campbell S, et al. A prospective, observational study of a chest pain observation unit in a British hospital. Emerg Med J 2002;19(2): 117–21.

69. Goodacre S, Nicholl J, Dixon S, et al. Randomised controlled trial and economic evaluation of a chest pain observation unit compared with routine care. BMJ 2004;328(7434):254.
70. Wiler JL, Ross MA, Ginde AA. National study of emergency department observation services. Acad Emerg Med 2011;18(9):959–65.
71. Baugh CW, Venkatesh AK, Bohan JS. Emergency department observation units: a clinical and financial benefit for hospitals. Health Care Manage Rev 2011; 36(1):28.
72. Venkatesh AK, Geisler BP, Chambers JJG, et al. Use of observation care in US emergency departments, 2001 to 2008. PLoS One 2011;6(9):e24326.
73. Baugh CW, Greenberg JO, Mahler SA, et al. Implementation of a risk stratification and management pathway for acute chest pain in the emergency department. Crit Pathw Cardiol 2016;15(4):131–7.
74. Bellew SD, Bremer ML, Kopecky SL, et al. Impact of an emergency department observation unit management algorithm for atrial fibrillation. J Am Heart Assoc 2016;5(2) [pii:e002984] Available at: https://www.ahajournals.org/doi/10.1161/JAHA.115.002984. Accessed November 2, 2019.
75. Southerland LT, Simerlink SR, Vargas AJ, et al. Beyond observation: protocols and capabilities of an emergency department observation unit. Am J Emerg Med 2018;37(10):1864–70. Available at: http://www.sciencedirect.com/science/article/pii/S0735675718310118. Accessed Novemeber 2, 2019.
76. Lo SM, Choi KTY, Wong EML, et al. Effectiveness of emergency medicine wards in reducing length of stay and overcrowding in emergency departments. Int Emerg Nurs 2014;22(2):116–20.
77. McGrath J, LeGare A, Hermanson L, et al. The impact of a flexible care area on throughput measures in an academic emergency department. J Emerg Nurs 2015;41(6):503–9.
78. Garrett JS, Berry C, Wong H, et al. The effect of vertical split-flow patient management on emergency department throughput and efficiency. Am J Emerg Med 2018;36(9):1581–4.
79. Wallingford G, Joshi N, Callagy P, et al. Introduction of a horizontal and vertical split flow model of emergency department patients as a response to overcrowding. J Emerg Nurs 2018;44(4):345–52.
80. Doran KM, Colucci AC, Hessler RA, et al. An intervention connecting low-acuity emergency department patients with primary care: effect on future primary care linkage. Ann Emerg Med 2013;61(3):312–21.e7.
81. Kirkland SW, Soleimani A, Rowe BH, et al. A systematic review examining the impact of redirecting low-acuity patients seeking emergency department care: is the juice worth the squeeze? Emerg Med J 2019;36(2):97–106.
82. Cha WC, Shin SD, Song KJ, et al. Effect of an independent-capacity protocol on overcrowding in an urban emergency department. Acad Emerg Med 2009; 16(12):1277–83.
83. Murphy SO, Barth BE, Carlton EF, et al. Does an ED flow coordinator improve patient throughput? J Emerg Nurs 2014;40(6):605–12.
84. Fulbrook P, Jessup M, Kinnear F. Implementation and evaluation of a 'navigator' role to improve emergency department throughput. Australas Emerg Nurs J 2017;20(3):114–21.
85. Traub SJ, Saghafian S, Judson K, et al. Interphysician differences in emergency department length of stay. J Emerg Med 2018;54(5):702–10.e1.
86. Melnick ER, Szlezak CM, Bentley SK, et al. CT overuse for mild traumatic brain injury. Jt Comm J Qual Patient Saf 2012;38(11):483–9.

87. Sharp AL, Nagaraj G, Rippberger EJ, et al. Computed tomography use for adults with head injury: describing likely avoidable emergency department imaging based on the Canadian CT head rule. Acad Emerg Med 2017;24(1): 22–30.
88. Hodgson NR, Saghafian S, Mi L, et al. Are testers also admitters? Comparing emergency physician resource utilization and admitting practices. Am J Emerg Med 2018;36(10):1865–9.
89. Carnevale TJ, Meng D, Wang JJ, et al. Impact of an emergency medicine decision support and risk education system on computed tomography and magnetic resonance imaging use. J Emerg Med 2015;48(1):53–7.
90. Kadhim-Saleh A, Worrall JC, Taljaard M, et al. Self-awareness of computed tomography ordering in the emergency department. CJEM 2018;20(2):275–83.
91. Valtchinov VI, Ip IK, Khorasani R, et al. Use of imaging in the emergency department: do individual physicians contribute to variation? Am J Roentgenol 2019; 213(3):637–43.
92. Wolfe RE, Sanchez LD. Effect of emergency physician burnout on patient waiting times. Intern Emerg Med 2018;13(3):373–4.
93. De Stefano C, Philippon A-L, Krastinova E, et al. Effect of emergency physician burnout on patient waiting times. Intern Emerg Med 2018;13(3):421–8.
94. Tawfik DS, Profit J, Morgenthaler TI, et al. Physician burnout, well-being, and work unit safety grades in relationship to reported medical errors. Mayo Clin Proc 2018;93(11):1571–80.
95. Lu DW, Dresden S, McCloskey C, et al. Impact of burnout on self-reported patient care among emergency physicians. West J Emerg Med 2015;16(7): 996–1001.
96. Chung AS, Wong ML, Sanchez LD, et al. Research priorities for physician wellness in academic emergency medicine: consensus from the Society of Academic Emergency Medicine Wellness Committee. AEM Educ Train 2018;2: S40–7.
97. Persico N, Maltese F, Ferrigno C, et al. Influence of shift duration on cognitive performance of emergency physicians: a prospective cross-sectional study. Ann Emerg Med 2018;72(2):171–80.
98. Wong ML, Anderson J, Knorr T, et al. Grit, anxiety, and stress in emergency physicians. Am J Emerg Med 2018;36(6):1036–9.
99. Eng MS-B, Fierro K, Abdouche S, et al. Perceived vs. actual distractions in the emergency department. Am J Emerg Med 2019;37(10):1896–903. Available at: http://www.sciencedirect.com/science/article/pii/S0735675719300051. Accessed November 4, 2019.
100. Shanafelt TD, Dyrbye LN, Sinsky C, et al. Relationship between clerical burden and characteristics of the electronic environment with physician burnout and professional satisfaction. Mayo Clin Proc 2016;91(7):836–48.

Queuing Theory and Modeling Emergency Department Resource Utilization

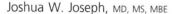

Joshua W. Joseph, MD, MS, MBE

KEYWORDS

• Emergency department operations • Throughput • Queueing • Efficiency

KEY POINTS

- Many different processes within the emergency department (ED) can be modeled using queueing equations, which can predict delays and help to identify bottlenecks to throughput.
- Average arrival times often hide variability that can significantly increase waiting times.
- As a resource approaches a utilization ratio of 1, waiting times for the resource grow dramatically.
- Although queueing equations can become mathematically complex, software packages that simulate queues help to predict the effects of changing resources in the ED without the need for tricky calculations.

INTRODUCTION

How many doctors does it take to manage the waiting room? It sounds like a simple question, which should have a simple answer, solved with algebra. An emergency physician (EP) can see X patients per hour. Y patients per hour arrive in the emergency department (ED). Should not the number of EPs needed to keep the waiting room clear be the number of patients who arrive per hour, divided by the number of patients per hour an EP can see?

The more one thinks about the problem, however, the more complex it becomes, and the less satisfactory the simplifying assumptions. Patients take different amounts of time to evaluate; a healthy 20 year old with a sore throat does not take the same amount of time as a 65 year old on dialysis presenting with fever and chest pain. Much also depends on the resources available to the ED, and the ED's current level of activity. If the ED has to share a computed tomography (CT) scan with the rest of the hospital, or if there is already a glut of samples at the laboratory, the EP

Department of Emergency Medicine, Beth Israel Deaconess Medical Center, Harvard Medical School, One Deaconess Road, Boston, MA 02215, USA
E-mail address: jwjoseph@bidmc.harvard.edu

Emerg Med Clin N Am 38 (2020) 563–572
https://doi.org/10.1016/j.emc.2020.04.006
0733-8627/20/© 2020 Elsevier Inc. All rights reserved.

can work flawlessly, but the number of patients in the waiting room will continue to grow.

This problem may have too many inputs and unknowns to be solved exactly, and variations within the workflow of the ED might lead two EDs with similar resources and patient volumes to different solutions. Yet, the question is too important to simply ignore or guess at. Staffing an ED has serious implications for its financial viability and for the safety and quality of care it delivers to its patients. It is also a question that has profound implications for the potential stresses and work-life balance issues that EPs and nurses may face, because the need to provide coverage for the ED at all times of day, every day of the year, imposes demands on their family life and circadian rhythms.

Thankfully, although we might not be able to create a perfect or exact answer to our question, we can make some important estimations. In the process, we can find out how to avoid several significant pitfalls that are commonly made by administrators when allocating resources in the ED. As the statistician George Box observed, "all models are wrong, but some are useful."[1]

MODELING RESOURCE USE AND STAFFING
Averages Are Not Enough

A simpler, related question to how many EPs are needed to staff an ED is how many nurses are needed to staff triage at a particular time. For most EDs, triage is a discrete process that takes a fixed amount of time. That the process is discrete means that we measure it in terms of individual patients, but for the purpose of modeling, we can also use discrete in the sense that triaging a patient is a self-contained process. The full patient evaluation conducted by an EP often contains many contingent stages, such as waiting for laboratory tests or imaging. Conversely, the typical steps of triage, such as identifying the patient, asking their chief complaint, obtaining vital signs, conducting a brief examination, and assigning a priority score (eg, ESI, ATS, or CTAS), are performed sequentially before seeing the next patient, and can be modeled as a single time period.[2–4]

A commonsense approach is to compare the average number of patients who arrive in the ED in a given period of time with the average number of patients that a nurse can triage in the same period of time. This makes some assumptions about the human factors involved, because we might be inclined to underestimate how quickly nurses can triage patients if some nurses can work faster under pressure for a period of time. However, obtaining a representative average that takes into account busy and calmer periods should help to even this out. Using this approach, an ED that averages 12 patients arriving per hour, where nurses can triage six patients per hour, would need two nurses to staff triage at a given time.

According to this approach, the two nurses intrepidly staffing the triage station should be ready to manage 12 patients per hour. Better yet, when the stars align and exactly 12 patients per hour arrive, our model suggests that as each patient arrives, one of the nurses will have just finished triaging the last arrival. Who would have thought that creating the "no wait" ED could be so simple.

Anyone who has worked in an ED knows that the results of this model do not match reality. However, it is difficult to explain exactly why this happens. It is tempting to accuse the averages of the time to triage a patient and the number of patients per hour of being misleading. Surely, our model hits a snag when the average underestimates the number of patients arriving per hour, and the waiting time builds up because during some hours the number of patients is higher than average, and perhaps there are times when our nurses are going more slowly.

Unfortunately, the averages are not really the problem; they remain an essential part of creating a representative model of an ED. Instead, the problem is in how we use the averages. We can make things even simpler, by imagining that in this ED, the average number of patients is ironclad, so that there are always 12 patients arriving per hour, and that the nurses always take 6 minutes to evaluate a patient. However, even in this imaginary ED, with triage staffed with two nurses, there will be times at which patients wait. Rarely, they may wait for a long time to be triaged. Even if our nurses become faster, or if we add a third nurse, it is still likely that some of the patients will have to wait.

The Problem of Arrivals and Variation

Waits arise in our ED because of variations in the amount of time between when patients arrive. If patients arrive at regularly spaced intervals (**Fig. 1**A), then they are triaged exactly as they arrive, and the arrivals perfectly match with the completion of the last patient's triage. However, variation in the amount of time between arrivals (**Fig. 1**B) means that there are idle periods in which one or more of the nurses does not have a new patient to triage, and unavoidable waiting periods in which a patient arrives while multiple nurses are already busy conducting a triage assessment.

Unlike when taking the average number of arrivals over a period of time, these losses of time do not even out. When a nurse is idle in triage and has no patient to see,

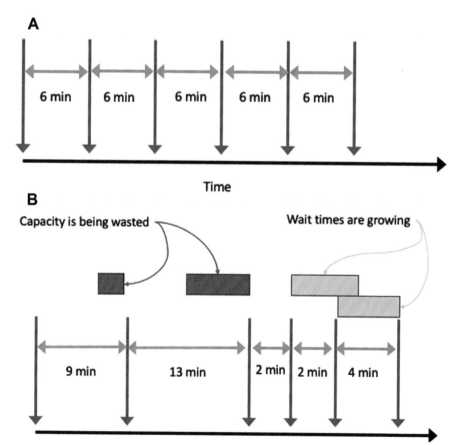

Fig. 1. (*A*) Regularly spaced arrivals; (*B*) Arrivals with typical variability.

they might be able to do something useful with that time, such as taking a break, going to the bathroom, or checking in with their colleagues. However, the only thing that they cannot do with the time they spend waiting to see a new patient is to use it to make up for future waits. There is no way to apply that time toward the patients who arrive when the nurses are busy; the amount of time they spend waiting simply accumulates, and can never be paid down.

When the variation between patient arrivals increases, the likelihood that patients will wait grows, as does the average amount of time they will wait. Although adding a third nurse at triage could certainly reduce these waits, doing so does not eliminate the potential for waits; it simply reduces them, because there could always be four patients who arrive in quick succession.

We can continue this process further as we add additional nurses, but doing so yields rapidly diminishing returns. Each additional nurse at triage is likely to spend a larger portion of their time waiting for a patient, because they will only be needed if a patient arrives while the preceding nurses are already busy. Using this strategy to staff our imaginary ED, which always sees six new patients an hour, means that the only way to ensure that patients never wait is to have six nurses at triage, one of whom will never see a patient unless all six of this hour's patients arrive in the same 10-minute period.

This becomes even less tenable once we start dealing with more realistic numbers of patients. If our six patients per hour really represents the average of a range from 1 patient per hour to 13, the potential costs of overstaffing become more glaring. Hospital management may want a "no wait" ED, but this is going to be a hard sell; we are better off trying to find if we can limit the amount of waiting to a degree that is feasible to staff and is still safe for our patients.

QUEUEING THEORY
What Is Queueing Theory?

Many of the pitfalls and tradeoffs that arise within these models are explained by queueing theory. Queueing theory is a branch of applied mathematics that is used to predict the behavior of lines (also known as queues), such as the length of a line over time, and the average time one spends waiting in a line. Although much of modern queueing theory emerged from the work of the Dutch mathematician A.K. Erlang, who used queueing models to predict the demand and use of telephone lines, it turns out that many of these properties apply no matter what the line is for. Queueing theory has been successfully applied across industries, streamlining services from manufacturing to airlines to restaurant service.[5-7]

Within the context of the ED, the same methodology is applied to model the queues for many different resources. Although there are slightly different assumptions that we need to make based on the kind of resource that we are modeling, the ways that the lines grow or shrink do not change. It does not matter whether the queues that we are concerned with are for physical resources, such as a CT scanner or laboratory tests, or for human resources, such as for registration clerks or for available nurses.

The mathematics involved in queueing analyses are sophisticated, but many of the lessons gained from even simple queueing models are useful to a broad variety of applications. You do not need to know the intricate details of queueing theory to reap many of its benefits. Furthermore, in day-to-day practice, many queueing models are approximated through the use of computer simulations and other programs that allow users to examine the behavior of underlying queues and the effects of changing their parameters, but without requiring the user to do the calculations themselves.

Little's Law

One of the most elementary theorems of queueing theory is Little's law.[8] Little's law states that the average size of a queue is proportional to the average rate of arrivals (usually referred to by the Greek letter λ), and the amount of time that a person spends in the queue.

L (average size of the queue) = λ (effective arrival rate) $\times$ W (average length of stay)

If an ED has an average arrival rate of six patients per hour, and the average patient has a length of stay of 3 hours, then Little's law dictates that the average occupancy of the ED will be 18 patients.[7,9]

Although Little's law is a fairly simple and intuitive equation, it actually took many years to prove conclusively. Little's law is a useful starting point for a queueing analysis because the formula is agnostic to how arrivals are distributed. If the average comes from patients being evenly distributed over time, or concentrated at any particular time interval (ie, if the patients mostly come at the end of the hour), then it still holds. We can also use Little's law for any portion of a larger system (we can apply Little's law to the ED directly, or we can apply it to any queue within the ED); it holds equally to describe the average occupancy of the ED, the average number of patients waiting for a CT scan, or any step of care that we choose.

Utilization

A direct result of Little's law, which provides a helpful understanding of the demand for a resource, is its utilization rate, commonly referred to by the Greek letter ρ. The utilization rate is the average patient arrival rate (λ) divided by the average service time (μ) for the resource. For instance, if a CT scanner receives four orders for CT scans per hour, and it can perform five scans per hour, then ρ of the CT scanner.

$\lambda/\mu = \rho$
is
$4/5 = 0.8$.

Although the utilization rate seems to only be a rearrangement of the terms from Little's law, it is useful because it provides a clear ratio of demand to capacity. If the utilization rate exceeds 1 at any point in time, then a backlog is guaranteed to develop and to continue getting worse. When accounting for increases in the variability of arrivals and service times, the ratio of utilization at which waits begin to grow rapidly may be considerably lower than one.

Kendall's Notation and Basic Queueing Models

Individual queues, which are used to examine any process within the ED, are frequently described using Kendall's notation.[5,10] Kendall's notation, typically in the form A/S/c, is a shorthand for describing the assumptions that underlie a queueing model. The "A" describes the arrival process (the pattern in which we assume patients arrive), "S" describes the service distribution (the pattern of how long it takes to provide a patient with a resource), and "c" refers to the number of servers (how many units of the resource we have). Fitting processes within the ED to these queueing models is helpful because some of them have closed form solutions, formulas that can reliably characterize how a process will perform over time.

A deterministic distribution, which has the notation "D," describes a process that occurs at a fixed rate. This is a reasonable description of some service distributions, but is generally a poor model for an arrival process. As we saw with the task of staffing triage, it is not particularly helpful to assume that patients arrive at a fixed rate.

However, some resources come close to always taking the same amount of time, such as a point-of-care blood glucose analyzer, which might be calibrated to take exactly 60 seconds for every sample. In Kendall's notation, our initial example, in which patients arrived at a fixed rate, and were triaged by two nurses who always took the same amount of time, would be known as a D/D/2 queue, because patients arrive at a determined rate, are served at a determined rate, and there are two nurses who provide the triage service.

A Markovian arrival process, which has the notation "M," has been shown in several studies to closely follow the arrival of the distribution of patient arrivals within EDs.[11–13] The most basic version of this process, the Poisson process, describes the time until the next patient arrives as an exponentially decreasing probability (**Fig. 2**). As a result, the average time between patient arrivals is often the balance point between "bursty" periods, where the interarrival times are short and several patients arrive in quick succession, and occasional long periods with no arrivals.

The simplest queue using this more rigorous model is the M/D/1 queue, which signifies patients arriving according to a Markovian arrival process, served by a single resource that follows a deterministic distribution. This model gives us a direct formula for the average time that a patient will need to wait in queue before they have access to the resource, which is:

Waiting time = ρ / 2μ $(1-\rho)$

If we imagine a single blood gas analyzer, which receives a new sample on average every 6 minutes (average arrival time λ = 10 specimen arrivals per hour), and takes 2 minutes to perform its analysis (average service time μ = 30 specimens analyzed per hour), with a utilization of ρ = 1/3, then our formula suggests that a specimen will sit for about 5 minutes before it is analyzed.

The M/M/1 and M/M/c queue models expand on this to reflect variation in the amount of time it takes to deliver a service. This makes it a much more suitable model for triage, because we can imagine that the average amount of time to perform triage reflects some cases where the process is quick and straightforward (an ankle sprain), virtually instantaneous (a patient with a prehospital ST-segment elevation myocardial infarction alert who is triaged at the bedside), or potentially long (a patient requiring a translator who cannot recall why they came to the ED). Accounting for this variation in the service effectively doubles our estimated wait time:

Waiting time = ρ / μ $(1-\rho)$

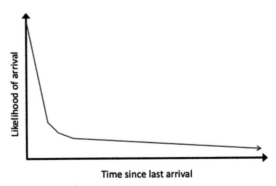

Fig. 2. The Poisson process graph.

Returning to our initial example of triage, with patients arriving every 6 minutes ($\lambda = 10$ patient arrivals per hour), and two nurses who each take on average 5 minutes to perform triage ($\mu = 12$ patients triaged per hour), leading to a utilization of $\rho = 10/12$, then our formula predicts that patients will wait an average of 25 minutes before they begin being triaged. If an extra patient comes every hour, our utilization increases to $\rho = 11/12$, and our average wait time before being triaged jumps to a painful 66 minutes.

As we approach a utilization of 1 in the M/M/c model, the average wait grows quickly (**Fig. 3**), without an appreciable bound. That the point of inflection in the curve shifts as the number of a resource increases is a direct result of the degree to which utilization changes.[14] If there are three nurses at triage rather than two, then every additional patient who arrives represents a proportionally smaller increase in utilization. Thus, when allocating a resource based on its expected utilization, it is extremely important to pay attention not only to the average utilization of the resource, but to how large surges in demand can be.

The M/D/1 and M/M/c models can also be used to calculate the likelihood of a certain number of patients being within a queue at a point in time, and the probability that a patient in the queue will wait for more or less than a specific amount of time.

RELATING QUEUEING THEORY TO PRACTICE
Ways to Get Around Increased Utilization

Many EDs experience periods when utilization exceeds a ratio of 1, and waits begin to spiral out of control. At those times, waits are typically reduced in a few different ways. The most problematic one is that initiated by patients: leaving without being seen. Although there are many factors that affect patients' decision to leave without being seen, the rate at which they do so is modeled using a queueing formula based on service rates in the ED as a whole.[15] Although the previously mentioned queueing formulas assume no upper limit on the number of potential patients waiting, more complex models exist that can account for the effects of limited capacity, and patients' decreasing willingness to wait as delays mount.

Some EDs have successfully addressed burgeoning waits by allowing flexible staffing patterns and care areas. In many EDs, some of these staffing policies exist on an informal basis. If triage is swamped, and few patients are being brought into treatment areas, more nurses may go to triage to help relieve their colleagues. In other EDs, dedicated fast track areas can be opened at periods of high demand, particularly if there are times of day in which there are higher volumes of patients with low-acuity presentations.[4,15–17]

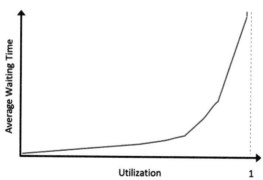

Fig. 3. Average wait time in the M/M/c model.

Similarly, some EDs have experimented with having lower-acuity patients schedule appointments within fast-track areas. Although the concept of an ED "appointment" may seem like a contradiction in terms, for urgent, but not necessarily emergent conditions that are not easily handled in a primary care office (eg, lacerations), this practice has merit. From a queueing theory standpoint, having patients schedule appointments, even if it is only an hour or two in advance, effectively turns their arrivals into a deterministic process, which can substantially reduce the amount of time they ultimately wait in queue.

A Successful Application of Queueing Theory in the Emergency Department

Perhaps the most successful application of queueing theory to ED operations was undertaken by Green and colleagues,[16] who used a series of M/M/c models to match the number of EPs on staff in a community hospital ED to match arrival rates at different times of day, factoring in a delay between the peak arrival rate in a given time period and the point at which it reached peak congestion. The study found that on days on which there was no change in the total number of physician hours, and hours were simply redistributed to better align with demand, there were substantial decreases in the number of patients who left without being seen, despite an increase in the overall volume of patients seen.

Can Getting Rid of the Waiting Room Speed up the Emergency Department?

The queueing models provide a mechanistic explanation for why waiting cannot be meaningfully eliminated in the ED, and unless an ED plans to let patients waiting to be seen line up outside, some kind of waiting room must remain. However, to the extent that "eliminating the waiting room," often refers to posting a physician at triage, it is an effective means of decreasing rates of patients leaving without being seen, and can decrease patients' overall length of stay.[17–19] Furthermore, the time patients spend in the waiting room before seeing a physician is often the kind of delay that they find most intolerable, making reducing this time a priority, even if overall delays are difficult to reduce.[20–22]

Posting a physician at triage is most appropriate for EDs that identify significant delays between patients completing triage and are brought back to a treatment space and evaluated by a physician. This is because of delays in patient transport, but is most commonly caused by crowding; a patient cannot be brought back if there is nowhere to bring them. This scenario is identified quickly by comparing the utilization of EPs relative to the utilization of triage. If the utilization of EPs is low, then moving the physician evaluation earlier in the process is probably worthwhile. If the utilization of EPs is already high, then moving physicians into triage may still reduce the left without being seen rate, but may not affect or even worsen some patients' length of stay.

Applying Queueing Theory to Everyday Emergency Department Operations

The performance of the ED itself reflects the interaction of multiple interlocking queues. A patient's evaluation and treatment will progress through triage and physician assessment, and can end there, or it can depend on several more queues, such as for laboratory tests, a CT scan, and an inpatient bed. The equations for the M/D/1 and M/M/c queues are powerful tools that can be used to analyze these processes and locate potential bottlenecks, which can cause a decrease in the utilization of processes elsewhere in the system. Multiple free online tools are available for analyzing basic queue models, including average waiting times and queues' probable occupancy (eg, https://www.supositorio.com/rcalc/rcalclite.htm and https://www.edqueue.org).

However, for the ED as a whole, no single set of equations can reliably predict the effects of changing a process on the system itself. Instead, software simulations are used to factor in the behavior of multiple queues over many trials and examine the effects of individual changes over time. Often, the process of improving the movement of a single queue within the ED, such as laboratory testing or imaging, can have significant downstream effects that simulation can effectively predict.[23–26] Simulation frameworks for queueing models are available as bespoke commercial applications (eg, ARENA, ProSim),[27] through packages for commercial software (eg, MATLAB), and as libraries for open-source software (eg, for C++ and Python).[28] Packages also exist for performing queueing analyses and simulations using commonly available spreadsheet software (eg, Microsoft Excel).

The prospect of modeling the operations of an entire ED may seem daunting, but the potential payoffs from applying queueing theory are immense. Occasionally a single bottleneck is critical to increased waits throughout the ED, even for patients who do not require its resources.[23] Although there exists no single solution to streamlining an ED, the application of queueing theory holds keys to identifying the most valuable targets for improvement, which remain unexplored in practice, despite a growing literature of simulation frameworks.[29–31] Whether these gains will ever be realized, however, remains in the hands of individual administrators.

DISCLOSURE

The author has nothing to disclose.

REFERENCES

1. Box GEP, Draper NR. Empirical model-building and response surfaces. Oxford (England): John Wiley & Sons; 1987. xiv, 669. (Empirical model-building and response surfaces).Introduction.
2. FitzGerald G, Jelinek GA, Scott D, et al. Emergency department triage revisited. Emerg Med J 2010;27(2):86–92.
3. Twomey M, Wallis LA, Myers JE. Limitations in validating emergency department triage scales. Emerg Med J 2007;24(7):477–9.
4. Wiler JL, Gentle C, Halfpenny JM, et al. Optimizing emergency department front-end operations. Ann Emerg Med 2010;55(2):142–60.e1.
5. Shortle JF, Thompson JM, Gross D, et al. Fundamentals of queueing theory. Hoboken, NJ: John Wiley & Sons; 2018. p. 566.
6. Takagi H. From computer science to service science: queues with human customers and servers. Comput Netw 2014;66:102–11.
7. Harris M. Little's law: the science behind proper staffing [Internet]. Emergency Physicians Monthly. 2010. Available at: https://epmonthly.com/article/littles-law-the-science-behind-proper-staffing/. Accessed November 17, 2019.
8. Little JDC. Little's law as viewed on its 50th anniversary. Oper Res 2011;59(3): 536–49.
9. Lovejoy WS, Desmond JS. Little's law flow analysis of observation unit impact and sizing. Acad Emerg Med 2011;18(2):183–9.
10. Kendall DG. Stochastic processes occurring in the theory of queues and their analysis by the method of the imbedded Markov chain. Ann Math Stat 1953; 24(3):338–54.
11. Armony M, Israelit S, Mandelbaum A, et al. On patient flow in hospitals: a data-based queueing-science perspective. Stoch Syst 2015;5(1):146–94.

12. Whitt W, Zhang X. A data-driven model of an emergency department. Oper Res Health Care 2017;12:1–15.
13. Kim S-H, Whitt W. Are call center and hospital arrivals well modeled by nonhomogeneous Poisson processes? Manuf Serv Oper Manag 2014;16(3):464–80.
14. Millsap C. Thinking clearly about performance. Queue 2010;8(9):10.
15. Wiler JL, Bolandifar E, Griffey RT, et al. An emergency department patient flow model based on queueing theory principles. Acad Emerg Med 2013;20(9): 939–46.
16. Green LV, Soares J, Giglio JF, et al. Using queueing theory to increase the effectiveness of emergency department provider staffing. Acad Emerg Med 2006; 13(1):61–8.
17. Abdulwahid MA, Booth A, Kuczawski M, et al. The impact of senior doctor assessment at triage on emergency department performance measures: systematic review and meta-analysis of comparative studies. Emerg Med J 2016;33(7):504–13.
18. Imperato J, Morris DS, Binder D, et al. Physician in triage improves emergency department patient throughput. Intern Emerg Med 2012;7(5):457–62.
19. Zayas-Caban G, Xie J, Green LV, et al. Policies for physician allocation to triage and treatment in emergency departments. IISE Trans Healthc Syst Eng 2019;0(0):1–15.
20. Maister D. The psychology of waiting lines. In: Czepiel J, Solomon M, Surprenant C, editors. The service encounter. Lexington (MA): Lexington Books; 1985. p. 113–23.
21. Soremekun OA, Takayesu JK, Bohan SJ. Framework for analyzing wait times and other factors that impact patient satisfaction in the emergency department. J Emerg Med 2011;41(6):686–92.
22. Dahlen I, Westin L, Adolfsson A. Experience of being a low priority patient during waiting time at an emergency department. Psychol Res Behav Manag 2012;5:1–9.
23. Storrow AB, Zhou C, Gaddis G, et al. Decreasing lab turnaround time improves emergency department throughput and decreases emergency medical services diversion: a simulation model. Acad Emerg Med 2008;15(11):1130–5.
24. Zeng Z, Ma X, Hu Y, et al. A simulation study to improve quality of care in the emergency department of a community hospital. J Emerg Nurs 2012;38(4):322–8.
25. Paul JA, Lin L. Models for improving patient throughput and waiting at hospital emergency departments. J Emerg Med 2012;43(6):1119–26.
26. Hung GR, Whitehouse SR, O'Neill C, et al. Computer modeling of patient flow in a pediatric emergency department using discrete event simulation. Pediatr Emerg Care 2007;23(1):5–10.
27. Wang T, Guinet A, Belaidi A, et al. Modelling and simulation of emergency services with ARIS and Arena. Case study: the emergency department of Saint Joseph and Saint Luc Hospital. Prod Plan Control 2009;20(6):484–95.
28. Dagkakis G, Heavey C. A review of open source discrete event simulation software for operations research. J Simul 2016;10(3):193–206.
29. Salmon A, Rachuba S, Briscoe S, et al. A structured literature review of simulation modelling applied to emergency departments: current patterns and emerging trends. Oper Res Health Care 2018;19:1–13.
30. Mohiuddin S, Busby J, Savović J, et al. Patient flow within UK emergency departments: a systematic review of the use of computer simulation modelling methods. BMJ Open 2017;7(5):e015007. Available at: https://bmjopen.bmj.com/content/7/5/e015007. Accessed November 15, 2019.
31. Hu X, Barnes S, Golden B. Applying queueing theory to the study of emergency department operations: a survey and a discussion of comparable simulation studies. Int Trans Oper Res 2018;25(1):7–49.

Factors Affecting Emergency Department Crowding

James F. Kenny, MD[a,*], Betty C. Chang, MD[a], Keith C. Hemmert, MD[b]

KEYWORDS

- Emergency department • Crowding • Boarding • Overcrowding • Throughput
- Operations

KEY POINTS

- Boarding of inpatients is one of the most significant causes of emergency department crowding.
- Emergency department boarding is the result of hospital-wide crowding and flow inefficiencies.
- Emergency department crowding and boarding have a negative impact across 7 key domains of emergency department administration and operations.
- Strategies to decrease emergency department crowding and boarding include microlevel (specific to the emergency department) or macrolevel (on a hospital- or health care system-wide scale) solutions.

INTRODUCTION

Emergency department (ED) crowding, sometimes referred to as overcrowding, has been identified as a barrier to timely and efficient care dating back to the 1980s.[1] Despite increased attention to this topic over the past 15 to 20 years, it continues to be a nearly ubiquitous and underappreciated public health crisis.[2] Although many factors contribute to crowding, boarding of inpatients has been found to be one of the most significant.[3] Boarding is the practice of keeping admitted patients in the ED for prolonged periods of time owing to insufficient inpatient capacity.[3–5] Boarding, and crowding as a whole, have adverse downstream effects on morbidity, mortality, patient satisfaction, and quality of care.[6] To develop sustainable solutions to crowding, it is essential to first understand its various causes and effects.

[a] Milstein Adult Emergency Department, NewYork-Presbyterian Hospital, Department of Emergency Medicine, Columbia University Irving Medical Center, 622 West 168th Street, Suite VC2-260, New York, NY 10032, USA; [b] Department of Emergency Medicine, Hospital of the University of Pennsylvania, Perelman School of Medicine at the University of Pennsylvania, 3400 Spruce Street, Ground Floor Ravdin, Philadelphia PA 19104, USA
* Corresponding author. 622 West 168th Street, Suite VC2-260, New York, NY 10032.
E-mail address: jfk2143@cumc.columbia.edu

Emerg Med Clin N Am 38 (2020) 573–587
https://doi.org/10.1016/j.emc.2020.04.001
0733-8627/20/© 2020 Elsevier Inc. All rights reserved.

emed.theclinics.com

HOW IS EMERGENCY DEPARTMENT CROWDING DEFINED AND MEASURED?

The American College of Emergency Physicians defines crowding as "a situation that occurs when the identified need for emergency services exceeds available resources for patient care in the ED, hospital, or both."[7] The inclusion of the "hospital" in this definition is key, because it highlights the fact that crowding is not an isolated ED issue, but rather a symptom of overall hospital and health care system crowding.[3,8] In the ED, this manifests in its most tangible form as boarding, which is why the 2 terms are often used synonymously.[1,3,4] Moreover, the concept of both ED and hospital processes contributing to crowding is reflected in commonly referenced crowding scoring systems, such as the National ED Overcrowding Scale.[1] Although measures such as ambulance diversion time, ED census, ED occupancy rate, and various boarding calculations have all been suggested and used as a means to measure this problem, there is still no gold standard measure of crowding.[9,10]

WHAT ARE THE CAUSES OF EMERGENCY DEPARTMENT CROWDING AND BOARDING?

For many years, high volumes of uninsured patients and patients with nonemergent issues were thought to be the primary sources of crowding, but this has since been refuted multiple times.[1,3,4] The causes of crowding are often categorized into 3 interdependent components that affect flow: input, throughput, and output (**Table 1**).[4,8,11,12] Table 1 describes the various factors that contribute to each of these 3 components, illustrating that the causes are multifactorial and complex.

Many of these factors are out of the ED's control. For instance, it is inherently difficult for the ED to control input factors, other than partnering with outpatient services or requesting ambulance diversion. To complicate matters, from the early 1990s to the late 2000s, the number of ED visits in the United States steadily increased, while the number of EDs and hospital beds decreased.[2,13,14] On the other end of the continuum, the fact that throughput depends on all output factors underscores the idea that ED flow depends on hospital flow.

For this reason, the input–throughput–output model is helpful not only for understanding ED flow and crowding, but also as a framework for conceptualizing hospital flow and capacity. It may be useful to think of the conceptual model in **Table 1** as a microlevel framework of patient crowding that only affects the ED, whereas the same conceptual model could be applied at a hospital or health care system level to understand the macrolevel input, throughput and output factors that lead to capacity and efficiency challenges impacting not just the ED, but every facet of the health care system.[1]

Boarding is the link between these 2 frameworks. Boarding patients affect ED throughput by consuming valuable resources such as space, the attention of staff, equipment, and diagnostic tests, limiting these resources for new ED patients.[4] Additionally, patients who board in the ED for prolonged periods of time actually have a longer hospital admission length of stay (LOS) than those who do not, perpetuating a vicious cycle of limited inpatient bed capacity and constrained output.[15,16] For this reason, we discuss potential solutions to boarding as a main factor in the ED crowding dilemma, while at the same time recognizing that it is not the only component.

WHAT ARE THE EFFECTS OF EMERGENCY DEPARTMENT CROWDING?

Research on the effects of ED crowding has increased in volume and quality for the past 20 years. The results show that crowding exerts negative effects on every aspect

Table 1
Causes of ED crowding

Component	Factors	Underlying Contributors
Input	Medical/surgical emergencies; urgent visits; nonurgent visits; ambulance arrivals; national "safety net"	Primary and urgent care capacity per hour of operation; outpatient referrals; nursing home referrals; mental health outpatient infrastructure; patient health insurance status; patient convenience; volume of surrounding hospitals; ambulance diversion of nearby hospitals; seasonal epidemics (ie, influenza)
Throughput	Patient acuity; triage and bed placement process; ED bed availability; staffing; diagnostic testing usage; degree of staff training and experience; consultant and ancillary services availability; degree of boarding	Aging population and patient complexity; laboratory and radiology turnaround times; inefficient bedding process; inefficient patient dispositions; inefficient ED operations and electronic medical record systems; all "output factors"
Output	Hospital occupancy; inpatient bed shortages; inpatient team "capping"; staffing ratios; inefficient processes of transferring care to inpatient team; skilled rehabilitation and nursing facility capacity; inefficient inpatient discharge planning; inpatient acuity; need to transfer to higher level of care	Elective surgical cases; inefficient surgical scheduling; transferred admissions from other hospitals; reservation or "holding" of inpatient beds for specific types of patients (ie, postoperative); sources of hospital revenue; defined nursing staffing ratios; decreased personnel on nights and weekends; insufficient resources such as telemetry

of care, even though the definition of crowding throughout this body of literature varies considerably. We categorize the effects of ED crowding into 7 domains (**Table 2**).

Operational Metrics

ED administrators as well as hospital executives have a keen interest in tracking operational metrics such as LOS for both ED and inpatient, wait times, and patients leaving without receiving the care they need (left without being seen and left before treatment complete). We consider time metrics here, and consider left without being seen and leave before treatment completion as access issues.

The epidemic of ED crowding is driven partially by increasing volumes across EDs nationally.[2,13,14] Volume increases are associated with higher overall LOS for both discharged and admitted patients, although it is interesting that the impact of volume increases varies depending on an ED's baseline volume (higher baseline volume EDs are better able to absorb an increase).[17,18]

As with other elements of crowding, ED boarding of inpatients is closely associated with a longer ED LOS for admitted and discharged patients.[19] Longer ED LOS is in turn linked with higher admission percentages, higher inpatient bed occupancy, and longer inpatient LOS.[17] Higher inpatient bed occupancy is also

Table 2
Key effects of ED crowding and main impacts

Domain	Impact of ED Crowding
Operational metrics	Longer ED LOS and longer inpatient LOS
Patient outcomes and adverse events	Increased mortality and medication errors
Quality measures	Worse performance on core CMS measures
Access to care	Higher LWBS, LBTC, and ambulance diversion
Patient experience	Worse Press Ganey and HCAHPS scores
Educational experience	Fewer patients and procedures for EM residents
Financial health	Significant financial losses for EDs and hospitals

Abbreviations: CMS, Centers for Medicare and Medicaid Services; EM, emergency medicine; HCAHPS, Health Care Providers and Systems; LBTC, leave before treatment completion; LWBS, left without being seen.

independently associated with longer ED LOS.[15–17,20,21] These 3 factors are linked in a negative feedback loop that can cause EDs and hospitals to operate with multiple inefficiencies.

Patient Outcomes and Adverse Events

ED crowding has been associated with a broad range of negative clinical outcomes for patients. In particular, crowding is associated with an increase in overall mortality rates,[21–25] and specifically with an increase in inpatient mortality among critically ill patients admitted via the ED.[26] ED crowding has also been linked to 7-day readmissions after ED discharge,[27] although this finding has been disputed[27,28] and seems to hinge on what measure of ED crowding is used. It should be noted that, although the literature is not uniform,[16] a preponderance of studies demonstrate this link. Patients who present to the ED with chest pain during times of high crowding have been shown to have a higher risk of adverse cardiovascular outcomes.[29] Finally, there is evidence that ED crowding is associated with increased rates of medication errors and other medical errors.[24,30,31]

Quality Measures

ED crowding has a negative impact on a number of core quality metrics.[32] In particular, an increase in LOS (again associated with ED crowding) is associated with an increased time to pain management for long bone fracture, a previously publicly reported Centers for Medicare and Medicaid Services metric.[33] ED crowding has also been linked to worse performance on Centers for Medicare and Medicaid Services quality measures for patients with community-acquired pneumonia,[24] longer time to critical therapies for patients with severe sepsis,[34] delays in assessment and treatment of pain,[35,36] delays in definitive therapy for acute myocardial infarction,[37,38] and decreased rates of hand hygiene.[39]

Access to Care

Access to care is a critical feature of EDs; it is valued by ED administrators as well as hospital executives. Access to care is typically proxied by rates of patients who walk out without getting the care they need (left without being seen and leave before treatment completion), as well as ambulance diversion hours.[40] High ED volumes and ED crowding have been linked with higher rates of patients who leave before treatment completion,[17] and higher probabilities of a patient leaving against medical advice, leaving without being seen, or leaving before treatment completion.[21,22,29,33]

Patient Experience

It is intuitive that ED crowding should be associated with lower patient satisfaction. This intuition is supported by a growing body of research: increased ED LOS is linked with a decrease in top box Press Ganey ratings for overall satisfaction and likelihood to recommend.[33,41] Patient dissatisfaction with ED crowding is not limited to discharged patients; ED crowding has also been shown to drive down patient satisfaction with inpatient stays.[41–43] It is not hard to imagine why this is: longer waits, less comfort, delays in care, and less privacy.[39,44,45]

Educational Experience

In the academic setting, crowding poses significant challenges to learners at all levels. During times of high ED crowding, emergency medicine residents see fewer patients and perform fewer procedures[46]; with crowding sustained at high levels, there is enormous educational impact throughout the course of a residency.[47] ED crowding is also the third most commonly reported source of dissatisfaction in a study of American emergency medicine residents' well-being.[48] ED crowding has also been shown to have an inverse relationship with medical students' performance on end-of-rotation examinations.[49]

Financial Health

Finally, ED crowding has a negative impact on the financial health of both the ED and the hospital. ED crowding is associated with increased costs for admitted patients,[23] as well as a loss in hospital revenue.[12,50] One study found that ED boarding increased costs by $6.8 million over 3 years.[51] Another found that decreasing boarding times by only 1 hour would increase revenue by $13,298 per day, or $4.9 million per year.[52] The negative financial implications for departments and hospitals are clear and can serve to jumpstart a discussion with hospital executives toward an institutional approach to this problem.

POTENTIAL SOLUTIONS TO EMERGENCY DEPARTMENT CROWDING: PATIENT FLOW STRATEGIES WITHIN A HEALTH CARE SYSTEM TO DECREASE EMERGENCY DEPARTMENT CROWDING AND BOARDING

As mentioned, ED patient flow revolves around a continuum of input, throughput, and output factors. Numerous improvement processes have been trialed and implemented to decrease ED crowding within this continuum of patient flow (**Table 3**). Some specific examples include (1) a split flow model, where patients with different acuity levels are funneled at intake to nonacute areas with better capacity to care for them efficiently (ie, fast track, provider-in-triage model, "vertical" midacuity area); (2) addressing throughput by tackling rate-limiting components of patient flow such as turnaround time for images, laboratory tests, and consults; and (3) off-loading patients from the ED to a separate acute care center (often known as an observation unit)—all with varying degree of success.[12,53–57]

The solution to ED crowding can also seem to be a classic supply and demand problem. If the number of patients arriving to an ED in any given day outpaces the ED's ability to bed and manage those patients, then the solution seems intuitive: increase bed and staffing capacity. Paradoxically, EDs that have increased their physical space have often found that it has not led to decreased crowding or improved

Table 3
Strategies to reduce ED crowding

	Component	Potential Solutions
Decrease demand	Input	Decreasing ED use (education/increase health literacy; access to primary care and specialty care)
		Addressing social determinants of health (housing, food, and utilities, uninsured patients, immigration, etc)
Increase capacity	Throughput	Staffing ratio (provider to RN, RN to patient)
		Aligning staffing with census and volume
		Intake models such as provider in triage and split flow (acute vs nonacute)
		Nurse-initiated protocols, standing orders
		Increasing resources and improving efficiency (turnaround for laboratory tests, imaging, consults, transport, float pool for nurses and ancillary staff during surge)
		Standardizing care on subgroup of patients (ie, geriatrics, mental health, pediatrics)
Increase capacity	Output	Macrolevel input solutions (**Table 4**)

operational metrics, and may actually making boarding worse.[58] These findings suggest that, in the case of the ED physical plant, size may not be the most important factor.

Given that ED boarding is a direct result of a demand and capacity mismatch within a hospital system, strategies to reduce boarding can be separated into microlevel approaches, which are specific to the ED, and macrolevel approaches, such as hospital bed capacity, infrastructure, and technological investments, as well as system-wide operations. The fact that multiple strategies inherent to the ED have had variable levels of success highlights that the key strategy to decrease ED crowding on a microlevel is to reduce ED boarding, that is, addressing the macrolevel problem.

What Are Some Potential Microlevel Strategies to Emergency Department Crowding and Boarding?

Evidence-based clinical pathways

Many EDs have instituted evidence-based clinical pathways to take care of unique cohorts of patients. These pathways help to standardize care and, for some subgroups, decrease admission rates.[59] Common clinical pathways revolve around diagnoses such as asthma, cellulitis, patients in stable vaso-occlusive crisis, chest pain, and lower risk syncope.[60,61] Standardization can also reduce excessive testing and admissions, that stem from fear of litigation and criticism by peers and patients.[62]

Embedding care coordination and patient navigation programs within the emergency department

Another strategy used with some success has been ED-embedded care coordination teams. EDs often serve as a safety net for patients who otherwise may not know how to navigate the complex medical system.[63] These hidden populations may also use the ED owing to a lack of access to care, poor health literacy, and even stigma.[64] In

Table 4
Strategies to reduce boarding and improve ED crowding

	Component	Potential Solutions
Decrease demand (microlevel)	Input	Evidence-based clinical pathways/standardization of care
		Embedding care coordination and patient navigation programs in the ED
		Robust outpatient linkage-to-care "follow-up" system
		Outpatient testing options
		Observation units/short stay units
		Medical home (hospital-at-home programs)
		Incorporating technology to enhance processes (digital health)
Increase capacity (macrolevel)	Throughput/output	Simplified admission process/established admission guidelines
		Centralized hospital-wide operations center
		Bed turnover, housekeeping, transport services
		Use of alcove and hallway beds
		Isolation cohorts
		Transferring certain cohorts of patients to affiliated hospital for inpatient care
		Routing elective and nonemergent workup to outpatient setting
		Embedding care coordination and patient navigation programs in inpatient setting
		Aligning education, clinical and operational missions in academic institutions
		Reverse triage for early discharges
		Standardization of care
		Discharge lounges, "get home safe" escort services, private ridesharing services
		Robust partnership with SNIFs, respite care, hospice programs
		Hospital-wide surge plan
		Rescheduling elective procedures
		Canceling outpatient clinics to bring in staff
		Postponing outpatient imaging
		Float pool of nurses and ancillary staff
		Cross-training and credentialing of staff (multihospital health care system)
		Hospital leadership commitment/institutional awareness
		Real-time flow dashboard
		A system of accountability
		Hospital-wide incentive programs for innovative initiatives targeting throughput

Abbreviation: SNIF, skilled nursing inpatient facility.

addition, EDs serve as a referral outlet for outpatient physicians who occasionally may not be available to their patients or feel their patient needs a higher level of care.

Some of the work of ED-based care managers and patient navigators includes assisting with linkage to care, preauthorization, and medication acquisition. They can also arrange for skilled nursing inpatient facility placement, home help, outpatient dialysis, and even nonemergent tests, thereby decreasing patient admissions. Health care system navigation programs and ED-based health educators can also play a role in community outreach, linkage to care, and patient education on health care resources.[65,66]

Robust outpatient long-term care systems and nonemergent testing options

These care management strategies can be paired with more robust outpatient linkage to care systems and nonemergent outpatient testing options. Although ED providers differ in practice style, experience, and risk aversion, developing a robust follow-up system that ensures patients get connected to outpatient services can help to decrease admissions by allaying concerns about discharging vulnerable patients who have poor access to outpatient services.[67]

In regard to outpatient testing, a multidisciplinary approach where radiology, ED, and outpatient clinics work together to establish continuation of care beyond ED is another potential way to reduce hospital admissions. Urgent imaging, such as MRI, echocardiography, and computed tomography scans, can be routed to outpatient diagnostic centers, thereby freeing up these services for truly emergent tests. Patients benefit by not taking on the costs and risks of a hospital admission while providers benefit from knowing that patients will receive needed imaging in a timely fashion.

Observation or short stay units

Other strategies that can impact hospital admissions are disposition pathways. These programs represent a bridge between microlevel and macrolevel factors because they lay at the intersection of ED and inpatient care.[68] One such strategy is building an observation unit or a short stay unit. After the initial evaluation and management in the ED, some patients may require additional time for evaluation and treatment, but not enough to warrant a full hospital admission. Rapid treatment and evaluation units or observation units fulfill this role by serving as an extension of treatment initiated in the ED. To decompress ED crowding, these units are often geographically separated from the ED.[69]

Certain illness and disease processes are highly conducive to observation admissions where objective criteria for risk stratification can help to streamline care. Conditions such as asthma, cellulitis, congestive heart failure, nonspecific abdominal pain, chest pain, and acute kidney injury have been shown to be safely managed within an observation setting, which can often avoid many of the time and staffing constraints of inpatient units.[60] Observation units can decrease ED boarding by moving a cohort of patients who would have otherwise occupied in-patient hospital beds to more temporary units, thus freeing up inpatient beds and resources for critically ill patients and ED beds for undifferentiated patients.[55,70]

Medical homes or hospital-at-home programs

Medical homes or hospital-at-home programs are another novel way to decrease overall hospital admissions. Here, select cohorts of patients are discharged home after their initial treatment in the ED. Patients can now stay in the comfort of their homes, while clinicians are deployed to continue the care.[71] The hospital may consider enacting a med-to-bed program to ensure that care is not interrupted during the peridischarge period. Medications that will be needed after the initial treatment are dispensed to patients at discharge.

Technological innovations such as telemedicine and continuous remote vital sign monitoring can enhance this alternative.[72] Using telemedicine, patients can be followed closely by a clinician after discharge from the ED, and can also receive other services remotely (consultants, care managers, social workers, etc). Although understudied, these hospital-at-home programs can likely decrease ED boarding by diverting less acute patients home while maintaining some of the benefits of an inpatient stay.

What Are Potential Macrolevel Approaches to Emergency Department Crowding and Boarding?

Simplified admission process

Admission processes should be simple and clear for more efficient throughput. Verbal handoffs between 2 attending physicians remains the gold standard for ensuring safety and smooth transitions, but can be difficult at times of rapid throughput or in academic institutions where there are trainees acting as the primary work force. Delays can be minimized if attending physicians are readily available regardless of who actually performs the handoff, should an issue arise.[73] Having a standardized admission process used by all inpatient services is another way to reduce delays and potentially maximize inpatient use.[73] In hospitals that have the capability, a standardized electronic signout process can allow for an efficient, asynchronous admission process, provided that attendings remain available to answer questions should they arise.

Efficient and active centralized hospital-wide operations center

Having a 24/7 centralized center for all admissions (both direct and indirect) can give an overall view of the state of the hospital, serving as a traffic control center. Efficient systems incorporate all aspects of patient flow, from input to output. This system should include bed turnover, housekeeping, and transport services.[74]

When there is a surge of admissions, the use of areas such as alcoves and hallways will increase capacity temporarily.[13] Cohorting patients with the same isolation status should also be considered. In a multihospital health system, transferring patients from the ED directly to an inpatient bed of an affiliated hospital for care is another alternative.[75]

Routing elective and nonemergent workup to outpatient setting

Given that the total inpatient LOS is tracked by Centers for Medicare and Medicaid Services, it is prudent to identify opportunities to mend factors that may delay a patient's discharge. Elective procedures as well as nonemergent imaging should be identified and routed to outpatient settings. Nonemergent consultations by specialists should also be arranged as outpatient.

Unless hospitals operate 24/7, the LOS will continue to grow. Reaching such an ideal state would likely put significant constraints on existing resources and staffing, and may be difficult to support financially by hospitals in the initial phase. However, this strategy to increase capacity is likely cost effective in the long term.[13] Hospitals may also consider establishing a robust outpatient network for tests, specialty clinics and follow-up care, as their first step.

Embedding care coordination and patient navigation programs within the hospital

This group of nonclinical staff facilitates patient flow. Described briefly earlier, their work begins even before admission by decreasing "avoidable" admissions.

Furthermore, this process can be most efficient if discharge planning begins the moment the patient is admitted. This multidisciplinary approach with continuous communication is key to early, safe discharges. This team should also include pharmacy, physical therapy/occupational therapy, clinical staff, family members, and patients.[76]

Aligning education, clinical, and operational missions in an academic institution

In academic institutions, where trainees serve as the primary care takers in the inpatient setting, there needs to be an alignment of trainee education and clinical responsibilities so that one does not compromise the other. In particular, the daily workflow cycle needs to be assessed so that early discharges are a priority for inpatient teams. Morning rounds can potentially be moved to evening rounds the evening before the anticipated day of discharge, so that patients can be discharged before noon, a critical time for arranging rehabilitation and other services.[77]

Reverse triage

Reverse triage is a process where patients who are stable and have the least need are expeditiously discharged.[78] Standardization of certain managements and the development of a minimal criteria for discharge can help to identify this cohort of patients. To increase bed availability, some hospitals have supplemented these processes by incorporating discharge lounges, get home safe patient escort programs, and partnership with private ridesharing services.[6] On the same token, established partnerships with skilled nursing inpatient facilities, rehabilitation centers, respite care, and hospice programs will also help to facilitate early discharges.

Adding a 24- to 48-hour postdischarge telemedicine follow-up with patients, along with the reverse triage and early discharge processes, can potentially bring a level of comfort to both providers and patients. Not only will this measure ensure patient safety, but it will also potentially improve the patient experience.[79]

Hospital-wide surge plans

In a crisis mode, where demand outweighs capacity of the hospital, clear actionable items by all services need to be in place to address boarding. Some examples include rescheduling elective procedures, canceling clinic appointments, bringing in staff to assist with inpatient care throughput, and postponing outpatient imaging so inpatient requests can be completed.[80]

Having a float pool of nurses and ancillary staff is not uncommon among large institutions. For smaller hospitals within a common health care system, cross-training and credentialing may be beneficial during times of surge. This strategy can also be an added benefit during system-wide mass casualty incident responses.[81]

Hospital leadership commitment and institutional awareness

Both microlevel and macrolevel approaches, as described elsewhere in this article, include some evidence-based strategies to address ED boarding. However, full hospital leadership support is essential to cultivate system-wide awareness and implement these strategies. The development of a real-time flow dashboard and a system of accountability may be of value.[82] Using evidence-based management tools such as lean six sigma and plan–do–study–act can further identify barriers.[83,84] A hospital-wide incentive program to foster innovative initiatives on patient throughput, can also be a way to increase awareness among different services and departments within the hospital.[3] Moreover, the introduction of timed patient disposition targets, through legislation, could push its resolution to the next level.[3]

SUMMARY

Understanding that the factors affecting ED crowding are part of a larger health care system-crowding problem is crucial to identifying the various adverse effects and exploring potential solutions. Boarding is one of the most substantial contributors to ED crowding, as well as one of the most appreciable markers of how hospital-wide crowding manifests in the ED.

Identified as a threat to public health more than 3 decades ago, the literature now supports the notion that crowding contributes to decreased quality of care and an increased strain on the overall health care system. Potential solutions, therefore, should continue to aim at comprehensive strategies that include the ED, hospital, overall health care system and public. Lastly, to effect change, the magnitude of this issue must first be understood and acknowledged by all stakeholders, so that accountability and sustainable solutions are established.

DISCLOSURE

The authors have nothing to disclose.

REFERENCES

1. Salway R, Valenzuela R, Shoenberger J, et al. Emergency Department (ED) over-crowding: evidence-based answers to frequently asked questions. Rev Médica Clínica Las Condes 2017;28(2):213–9.
2. Institute of Medicine. Hospital-based emergency care: at the breaking point. Washington, DC: The National Academies Press; 2007.
3. Rabin E, Kocher K, McClelland M, et al. Solutions to emergency department "boarding" and crowding are underused and may need to be legislated. Health Aff 2012;31(8):1757–66.
4. Government Accountability Office. Hospital emergency departments; crowding continues to occur, and some patients wait longer than recommended time frames. Washington, DC: GAO; 2009.
5. American College of Emergency Physicians (ACEP). Definition of Boarded Patient. Policy statement. Ann Emerg Med 2018;57(5):548.
6. Emergency Medicine Practice Committee, ACEP. Emergency department crowding: high impact solutions. 2016.
7. American College of Emergency Physicians (ACEP). Crowding. Policy statement. Ann Emerg Med 2013;61(6):726–7.
8. Rathlev NK, Chessare J, Olshaker J, et al. Time series analysis of variables associated with daily mean emergency department length of stay. Ann Emerg Med 2007;49(3):265–71.
9. Pines JM. Emergency department crowding in California: a silent killer? Ann Emerg Med 2013;61(6):612–4.
10. Solberg LI, Asplin BR, Weinick RM, et al. Emergency Department crowding: consensus development of potential measures. Ann Emerg Med 2003;42(6):824–34.
11. Asplin BR, Magid DJ, Rhodes KV, et al. A conceptual model of emergency department crowding. Ann Emerg Med 2003;42(2):173–80.
12. Hoot NR, Aronsky D. Systematic review of emergency department crowding: causes, effects, and solutions. Ann Emerg Med 2008;52(2):126–36.

13. Viccellio A, Santora C, Singer AJ, et al. The association between transfer of emergency department boarders to inpatient hallways and mortality: a 4-year experience. Ann Emerg Med 2009;54(4):487–91.

14. Sayah A, Rogers L, Devarajan K, et al. Minimizing ED waiting times and improving patient flow and experience of care. Emerg Med Int 2014;2014:1–8.

15. Nippak PMD, Isaac WW, Ikeda-Douglas CJ, et al. Is there a relation between emergency department and inpatient lengths of stay? Can J Rural Med 2014; 19(1):12–20.

16. Derose SF, Gabayan GZ, Chiu VY, et al. Emergency department crowding predicts admission length of-stay but not mortality in a large health system. Med Care 2014;52(7):6002–611.

17. Handel DA, Fu R, Vu E, et al. Association of emergency department and hospital characteristics with elopements and length of stay. J Emerg Med 2014;46(6): 839–46.

18. Handel DA, Sun B, Augustine JJ, et al. Association among emergency department volume changes, length of stay, and leaving before treatment complete. Hosp Top 2015;93(3):53–9.

19. White BA, Biddinger PD, Chang Y, et al. Boarding inpatients in the emergency department increases discharged patient length of stay. J Emerg Med 2013; 44(1):230–5.

20. Verelst S, Wouters P, Gillet JB, et al. Emergency department crowding in relation to in-hospital adverse medical events: a large prospective observational cohort study. J Emerg Med 2015;49(6):949–61.

21. Singer AJ, Thode HC, Viccellio P, et al. The association between length of emergency department boarding and mortality. Acad Emerg Med 2011;18(12): 1324–9.

22. Bernstein SL, Aronsky D, Duseja R, et al. The effect of emergency department crowding on clinically oriented outcomes. Acad Emerg Med 2009;16(1):1–10.

23. Sun BC, Hsia RY, Weiss RE, et al. Effect of emergency department crowding on outcomes of admitted patients. Ann Emerg Med 2013;61(6).

24. F. George, K. Evridiki, The Effect of Emergency Department Crowding on Patient Outcomes, Health Sci. J 9 (1), 2015, 1-6.

25. Jo S, Jin YH, Lee JB, et al. Emergency department occupancy ratio is associated with increased early mortality. J Emerg Med 2014;46(2):241–9.

26. Jo S, Jeong T, Jin YH, et al. ED crowding is associated with inpatient mortality among critically ill patients admitted via the ED: post hoc analysis from a retrospective study. Am J Emerg Med 2015;33(12):1725–31.

27. Gabayan GZ, Derose SF, Chiu VY, et al. Emergency department crowding and outcomes after emergency department discharge. Ann Emerg Med 2015;66(5): 483–92.e5.

28. Hsia RY, Asch SM, Weiss RE, et al. Is emergency department crowding associated with increased "bounceback" admissions? Med Care 2013;51(11):1008–14.

29. Pines JM, Pollack CV, Diercks DB, et al. The association between emergency department crowding and adverse cardiovascular outcomes in patients with chest pain. Acad Emerg Med 2009;16(7):617–25.

30. ED overcrowding is associated with an increased frequency of medication errors. In: Kulstad EB, Sikka R, Sweis RT, et al, editors. Am J Emerg Med 2010;28(3): 304–9.

31. Epstein SK, Huckins DS, Liu SW, et al. Emergency department crowding and risk of preventable medical errors. Intern Emerg Med 2012;7(2):173–80.

32. Moskop JC, Geiderman JM, Marshall KD, et al. Another look at the persistent moral problem of emergency department crowding. Ann Emerg Med 2018; 74(3):357–64.

33. Chang AM, Lin A, Fu R, et al. Associations of emergency department length of stay with publicly reported quality-of-care measures. Acad Emerg Med 2017; 24(2):246–50.

34. Gaieski DF, Agarwal AK, Mikkelsen ME, et al. The impact of ED crowding on early interventions and mortality in patients with severe sepsis. Am J Emerg Med 2017; 35(7):953–60.

35. Pines JM, Shofer FS, Isserman JA, et al. The effect of emergency department crowding on analgesia in patients with back pain in two hospitals. Acad Emerg Med 2010;17(3):276–83.

36. Mills AM, Shofer FS, Chen EH, et al. The association between emergency department crowding and analgesia administration in acute abdominal pain patients. Acad Emerg Med 2009;16(7):603–8.

37. Kulstad EB, Kelley KM. Overcrowding is associated with delays in percutaneous coronary intervention for acute myocardial infarction. Int J Emerg Med 2009;2(3): 149–54.

38. Ward MJ, Baker O, Schuur JD. Association of emergency department length of stay and crowding for patients with ST-elevation myocardial infarction. West J Emerg Med 2015;16(7):1067–72.

39. Chang BP, Carter E, Suh EH, et al. Patient treatment in ED hallways and patient perception of clinician-patient communication. Am J Emerg Med 2016;34(6): 1163–4.

40. Hsia RY, Sarkar N, Shen YC. Is inpatient volume or emergency department crowding a greater driver of ambulance diversion? Health Aff 2018;37(7): 1115–22.

41. Wang H, Kline JA, Jackson BE, et al. The role of patient perception of crowding in the determination of real-time patient satisfaction at Emergency Department. Int J Qual Health Care 2017;29(5):722–7.

42. Tekwani KL, Kerem Y, Mistry CD, et al. Emergency department crowding is associated with reduced satisfaction scores in patients discharged from the emergency department. West J Emerg Med 2013;14(1):11–5.

43. Lin YK, Lin CJ. Factors predicting patients' perception of privacy and satisfaction for emergency care. Emerg Med J 2011;28(7):604–8.

44. Lin YK, Lee WC, Kuo LC, et al. Building an ethical environment improves patient privacy and satisfaction in the crowded emergency department: a quasi-experimental study. BMC Med Ethics 2013;14(1):8.

45. Stoklosa H, Scannell M, Ma Z, et al. Do EPs change their clinical behaviour in the hallway or when a companion is present? A cross-sectional survey. Emerg Med J 2018;35(7):406–11.

46. Mahler SA, McCartney JR, Swoboda TK, et al. The impact of emergency department overcrowding on resident education. J Emerg Med 2012;42(1):69–73.

47. Atzema C, Bandiera G, Schull MJ, et al. Emergency department crowding: the effect on resident education. Ann Emerg Med 2005;45(3):276–81.

48. Perina DG, Marco CA, Smith-Coggins R, et al. Well-Being among emergency medicine resident physicians: results from the ABEM longitudinal study of emergency medicine residents. J Emerg Med 2018;55(1):101–9.e2.

49. Wei G, Arya R, Trevor Ritz Z, et al. How does emergency department crowding affect medical student test scores and clerkship evaluations? West J Emerg Med 2015;16(6):913–8.

50. Bayley MD, Schwartz JS, Shofer FS, et al. The financial burden of emergency department congestion and hospital crowding for chest pain patients awaiting admission. Ann Emerg Med 2005;45(2):110–7.

51. Krochmal P, Riley TA. Increased health care costs associated with ED overcrowding. Am J Emerg Med 1994;12(3):265–6.

52. Pines JM, Batt RJ, Hilton JA, et al. The financial consequences of lost demand and reducing boarding in hospital emergency departments. Ann Emerg Med 2011;58(4):331–40.

53. Love RA, Murphy JA, Lietz TE, et al. The effectiveness of a provider in triage in the emergency department: a quality improvement initiative to improve patient flow. Adv Emerg Nurs J 2012;34(1):65–74.

54. Arya R, Wei G, Mccoy JV, et al. Decreasing length of stay in the emergency department with a split emergency severity index 3 patient flow model. Acad Emerg Med 2013. https://doi.org/10.1111/%28ISSN%291553-2712/homepage/ForAuthors.html.

55. Baugh CW, Venkatesh AK, Bohan JS. Emergency department observation units: a clinical and financial benefit for hospitals. Health Care Manage Rev 2011;36(1):28–37.

56. Towbin AJ, Iyer SB, Brown J, et al. Practice policy and quality initiatives: decreasing variability in turnaround time for radiographic studies from the emergency department. Radiographics 2013;33(2):361–71.

57. Holland LL, Smith LL, Blick KE. Reducing laboratory turnaround time outliers can reduce emergency department patient length of stay: an 11-hospital study. Am J Clin Pathol 2005;124(5):672–4.

58. Mumma BE, McCue JY, Li CS, et al. Effects of emergency department expansion on emergency department patient flow. Acad Emerg Med 2014;21(5):504–9.

59. Di Somma S, Paladino L, Vaughan L, et al. Overcrowding in emergency department: an international issue. Intern Emerg Med 2015;10(2):171–5.

60. Rutman L, Migita R, Spencer S, et al. Standardized asthma admission criteria reduce length of stay in a pediatric emergency department. Acad Emerg Med 2016;23(3):289–96.

61. Yarbrough PM, Kukhareva PV, Spivak ES, et al. Evidence-based care pathway for cellulitis improves process, clinical, and cost outcomes. J Hosp Med 2015;10(12):780–6.

62. Kanzaria HK, Hoffman JR, Probst MA, et al. Emergency physician perceptions of medically unnecessary advanced diagnostic imaging. Acad Emerg Med 2015;22:390–8.

63. Tricco AC, Antony J, Ivers NM, et al. Effectiveness of quality improvement strategies for coordination of care to reduce use of health care services: a systematic review and meta-analysis. CMAJ 2014;186(15):E568–78.

64. Maldonado CZ, Rodriguez RM, Torres JR, et al. Fear of discovery among Latino immigrants presenting to the emergency department. Acad Emerg Med 2013;20(2):155–61.

65. Enard KR, Ganelin DM. Reducing preventable emergency department utilization and costs by using community health workers as patient navigators. J Healthc Manag 2013;58(6):412–27.

66. Lowthian JA, Smith C, Stoelwinder JU, et al. Why older patients of lower clinical urgency choose to attend the emergency department. Intern Med J 2013;43(1):59–65.

67. Chou SC, Deng Y, Smart J, et al. Insurance status and access to urgent primary care follow-up after an emergency department visit in 2016. Ann Emerg Med 2018;71(4):487–96.
68. Martinez E, Reilly BM, Evans AT, et al. The observation unit: a new interface between inpatient and outpatient care. Am J Med 2001;110(4):274–7.
69. Lee IH, Chen CT, Lee YT, et al. A new strategy for emergency department crowding: high-turnover utility bed intervention. J Chin Med Assoc 2017;80(5):297–302.
70. Konnyu KJ, Kwok E, Skidmore B, et al. The effectiveness and safety of emergency department short stay units: A rapid review. Open Med 2012;6(1):10–6.
71. Shepperd S, Iliffe S, Ha D, et al. Admission avoidance hospital at home (Review) summary of findings for the main comparison. 2016;(9). https://doi.org/10.1002/14651858.CD007491.pub2.www.cochranelibrary.com
72. De San Miguel K, Smith J, Lewin G. Telehealth remote monitoring for community-dwelling older adults with chronic obstructive pulmonary disease. Telemed E-health 2013;19(9):652–7.
73. Kelen GD. Hospital and emergency department crowding impact on patient-centered care and suggested solutions. Hopkins Med J 2013.
74. Lovett PB, Illg ML, Sweeney BE. A successful model for a comprehensive patient flow management center at an academic health system. Am J Med Qual 2014;31(3):246–55.
75. Nezamoddini N, Khasawneh MT. Modeling and optimization of resources in multi-emergency department settings with patient transfer. Oper Res Heal Care 2016;10:23–34.
76. Plant N, Mallitt KA, Kelly PJ, et al. Implementation and effectiveness of "care navigation", coordinated management for people with complex chronic illness: rationale and methods of a randomised controlled. BMC Health Serv Res 2013;13(1):1–6.
77. Wertheimer B, Jacobs REA, Bailey M, et al. Discharge before noon: an achievable hospital goal. J Hosp Med 2014;9(4):210–4.
78. Pollaris G, Sabbe M. Reverse triage: more than just another method. Eur J Emerg Med 2016;23(4):240–7.
79. Morrissey J. Hospitals seek solutions for patient transportation. Health Progress 2019;100(5).
80. Sheikhbardsiri H, Raeisi AR, Nekoei-moghadam M, et al. Surge capacity of hospitals in emergencies and disasters with a preparedness approach: a systematic review. Disaster Med Public Health Prep 2017;11(5):612–20.
81. Adalja AA, Watson M, Bouri N, et al. Absorbing citywide patient surge during Hurricane Sandy: a case study in accommodating multiple hospital evacuations. Ann Emerg Med 2014;64(1):66–73.e1.
82. Chang AM, Cohen DJ, Lin A, et al. Hospital strategies for reducing emergency department crowding: a mixed-methods study. Ann Emerg Med 2018;71(4):497–505.e4.
83. Holden RJ. Lean thinking in emergency departments: a critical review. Ann Emerg Med 2011;57(3):265–78.
84. Maxey M, editor. The lean six sigma pocket toolbook a quick reference guide to nearly 100 tools for improving process quality, speed, and complexity. New York: McGraw-Hill; 2005.

Staffing and Provider Productivity in the Emergency Department

Bryan A. Stenson, MD[a],*, Jared S. Anderson, MD[b],
Samuel R. Davis, PhD[c]

KEYWORDS

- Productivity • Staffing • Scheduling • Rostering • Capacity • Demand • Staircase

KEY POINTS

- Managing productivity and staffing in the emergency department is an ongoing journey, not a static destination.
- Data collection and metrics are critical for identifying improvement opportunities.
- The emergency department is a system within a system of systems; communication and coordination with other departments are critical to extract the maximum benefit from emergency department operations.
- A thorough understanding of demand and capacity allows for meaningful scheduling adjustments to improve throughput and the overall provider experience.
- Provider productivity is not static; it decreases in a stepwise manner over the course of a shift. Staffing based on this "staircase" model permits more accurate measures of demand and capacity.

INTRODUCTION

Staffing and productivity are at the core of any efficient emergency department (ED). Appropriate staffing increases throughput, lowers departmental costs, and improves flow. Understanding the drivers of productivity can allow managers to maximize providers' efficiency and measure workload.

Although this article focuses on variables more directly in the control of departmental leadership, skilled leaders must understand that both staffing and productivity have significant interplay with factors beyond the control of ED staff. These factors include—but are not limited to—overall volume, patient acuity, crowding, and other linked processes such as nursing, radiology, laboratories, and inpatient bed availability.

[a] Beth Israel Deaconess Medical Center, Harvard Medical School, One Deaconess Road, Boston, MA 02215, USA; [b] Brown University School of Medicine, Brown Emergency Medicine, 55 Claverick Street Floor 2, Providence, RI 02903, USA; [c] Northeastern University, 334 Snell Engineering Center, Boston, MA 02115, USA
* Corresponding author.
E-mail address: bstenson@bidmc.harvard.edu

Emerg Med Clin N Am 38 (2020) 589–605
https://doi.org/10.1016/j.emc.2020.04.002
0733-8627/20/© 2020 Elsevier Inc. All rights reserved.
emed.theclinics.com

Significant research has been performed to assess factors that affect the productivity of attending emergency physicians—ranging from the impact of scribes to appropriate shift lengths—although such studies are still underrepresented within the broader discourse of emergency medicine research. By providing a readily available summary of these findings, we offer guidance to help increase productivity within individual EDs' unique limitations.

The foundations of staffing are simple for smaller EDs where single coverage is sufficient throughout the day. As volume increases, the complexity of staffing options increases. Decisions include adding attending physicians and advanced practice practitioners (APPs), as well as changes to shift length, timing, and the degree of overlap. This section discusses tools to handle the first few tiers of complexity in a stepwise manner.

PRODUCTIVITY
Measuring Productivity

Despite being an essential element of ED management, there exists no standard productivity measure for emergency physicians. Productivity is most commonly defined as the ability of an attending physician to see, treat, and disposition new patient arrivals. The most frequently used individual measurements are the number of patients seen per hour and the relative value units (RVUs) a physician generates per hour. Both metrics quantify the work completed over time, although only the second incorporates patient complexity. Measuring RVUs per patient has distinct advantages, because it is often linked directly to billing and helps to control for case complexity (**Table 1**). A 2012 survey of department chairs showed the majority tracked productivity to determine compensation.[1] Although RVUs were the most common metric for incentivizing physicians, other factors include patient satisfaction, length of stay metrics, publications, grants, and committee attendance. Unfortunately, neither patients seen nor RVUs generated per hour are perfect measures, because they exclude time spent after assigned shifts seeing patients and documenting, time spent on signed out cases, and other unmeasured contributions to patient care.

Table 1		
Pros and cons of common productivity metrics		
Metric	**Pros**	**Cons**
Patients per hour	Easy information to gather Correlates with capacity planning	Does not account for patient acuity Does not account for departmental issues (crowding, etc) May incentivize cherry picking of patients likely to have low complexity
RVUs per hour	Correlates to revenue Incorporates both complexity and volume	Cannot calculate until billing information is complete Does not account for departmental issues (crowding, etc) May incentivize cherry picking of patients likely to have high RVU reimbursement
RVUs per patient	Encourages capturing appropriate complexity and charting	Depends on thoroughness of charting May incentivize additional testing and procedures on patients Does not encourage department throughput

Drivers of Productivity

Prior research shows that both attending and resident productivity follows a predictable hourly decrease throughout a shift.[2,3] Providers start a shift operating at their highest productivity level with a stepwise decrease as the shift progresses, forming a staircase shape. Signed out patients without clear dispositions have a notable effect on productivity.[4] In this section, we review the roles and processes that have been demonstrated to have effects on ED productivity.

Roles

The presence of a variety of different roles in the ED—both providers and nonproviders—has been studied to determine the effects of productivity (**Table 2**).

Advanced practice practitioners Data on the overall benefits of APPs is limited, but suggests that they can be a potent addition to productivity in certain clinical contexts. When compared with resident physicians, APPs were found to see more patients per hour and generate more RVUs per hour than resident physicians—an average of 2.21 relative to 1.53 patients per hour.[5] This difference may be due to experience; by definition, residents have been working for a few years at most, whereas many APPs' experience may come primarily from seeing lower acuity complaints. A potentially fraught productivity benefit of APPs staffing versus trainees is that, in many EDs, APPs do not necessarily staff lower acuity patients with a supervising physician, which may intrigue some administrators while causing heartburn for others.

Another study by the same group found that, even in higher acuity settings, APPs still see slightly more patients per hour than residents.[6] However, in these settings a resident actually generates more RVUs per hour, because APPs may still tend to see lower acuity patients within the setting, and residents conversely tend to document more thoroughly.

Resident physicians Residents are an integral part of the staffing of most academic medical centers, but are also present within many community hospital EDs to varying degrees. Among the most substantial distinctions between residents are whether they are EM trainees or off service from other specialties. Off-service residents tend to see fewer patients per hour than emergency medicine residents,[3,7,8] and even direct interventions to motivate and track off-service residents' patient encounters have only been shown to minimally increase their productivity.[9]

The productivity of emergency medicine residents increases markedly during training, with the greatest gains in patients per hour and RVUs per hour occurring

Table 2 Common ED roles	
Role	**Key Points**
APPs	Productivity difficult to measure; have both independent productivity (unstaffed low acuity cases) and dependent productivity (staffed cases) Excel in certain settings (eg, fast track)
Residents	Have no true independent productivity (attending must staff) Increase attending productivity and complicate its measurement Administrators have limited control over resident staffing Vary in training background and experience level
Students	Generally do not increase or decrease attending or resident productivity
Scribes	Off-load various tasks to allow for increased productivity

between the first and second years of training.[8,10–13] The data for postgraduate year 3 and postgraduate year 4 residents is somewhat limited because senior residents serve in supervisory or teaching roles at many academic sites and perform other non–RVU-generating activities.[10] How more advanced trainees perform within community ED rotations and while moonlighting requires further investigation, but likely approaches that of attending physicians.

Although there has long been a perception that teaching slows down clinical care, several studies have demonstrated that the presence of EM residents positively impacts attending productivity. In one instance, the creation of an EM residency increased attending RVUs per hour by 4.98. As each class was added, RVUs per hour increased in a stepwise manner. Overall, 32% more patients would be seen, and staffing hours decreased by 6% for attending physicians and 60% for APPs.[14] However, any savings from a new residency program need to be balanced against the substantial costs of time and resources outside of the clinical sphere. For departments with existing programs, residents have been shown to increase the number of patients per hour by 0.12 versus attending-only shifts.[15,16]

Medical students Although medical students are just starting their medical education, cannot work independently, and require more intensive supervision than residents, the literature suggests that these factors likewise do not have a negative impact on productivity. When medical students are present and supervised by residents, they do not have a negative impact on residents' patients per hour or RVUs per hour.[17] Unlike residents, medical students did not lead to increased attending productivity or changes in throughput times.[15,16] Although there may be other qualitative factors involved in working with medical students (perhaps attending physicians simply work harder in their presence), they should not be regarded as an operational resource in terms of increasing productivity in an ED.

A controversial topic related to productivity is the effect that dedicated teaching has on productivity. Many studies cite a commonly held belief that teaching demands while working clinically decreases overall productivity. This effect has not been demonstrated consistently. Multiple studies looked at whether higher RVUs per hour are associated with lower median teaching evaluations and no correlation was found.[18–20] In fact, higher teaching performance ratings were found to be associated with more RVUs per hour.[21] Structured interviews with these high-performing providers found they focused on seeing a high volume of patients, dictating each one immediately, and focusing on a teaching point for each case. So, although this belief is commonly held, there has been no documented negative relationship between quality of teaching and overall department productivity.

Scribes Scribes have the potential to provide productivity gains across a variety of domains. Although they are primarily known for facilitating charting on shift, they may help with a variety of tasks, such as following up on laboratory tests and sending pages. Several studies have demonstrated significant gains in productivity from employing scribes, ranging from to 0.8 patients per hour and 2.4 RVUs per hour over a 10-hour shift when working with scribes,[22,23] with increase of 0.15 RVUs per patient, likely owing to improved billing from documentation. Notably, the quality of scribes' documentation has not been studied extensively, which is needed to better understand the nature of this effect on RVUs per patient.[24] Although some of the productivity benefits of scribes may accrue from their ability to help physicians to mitigate some of the inefficiencies of electronic health records, there are also likely important qualitative benefits that scribes may offer emergency physicians, such as increased time spent at the bedside or increased availability to teach. Ultimately, the benefits of a scribe program must be balanced against its hourly and administrative costs.

Processes

Shift length The most common shift lengths of 8 and 12 hours carry unique trade-offs.[25] Both lengths can have an impact on circadian scheduling, but the fatigue in the last few hours of a 12-hour shift has the potential to coincide with the existing decrease in new patients seen per hour found in the staircase model. For emergency medicine residents, working 9-hour shifts has been shown to lead residents to naturally assume a higher overall rate of patients per hour than those working 12-hour shifts.[26] Shift length also has implications beyond individual provider productivity; shorter shifts also allow for more flexibility to increase staffing during high-volume periods.

However, despite the potential productivity benefits of shorter shifts, longer shifts are the most viable option for low-volume centers with few providers on staff. Similarly, longer shifts may be preferred by groups who wish to work fewer shifts overall, because they allow fewer providers to work during undesirable times, such as nights, weekends, and holidays.

Shift overlap and sign-outs The goal of overlapping shifts is to provide a dedicated time for the outgoing provider to clean up his or her patients so that the oncoming provider will have less to do for each signed-out patient. This is another potential disadvantage of longer (eg, 12-hour) shifts, although the prospect of adding an hour of explicit overlap to an 8-hour shift, during which no new patients are seen, is much more palatable. However, studies examining overlap note that the practice does not necessarily lead to significantly fewer signed-out patients,[27] although these patients may require less additional work on the part of the oncoming provider. Comparatively, the waterfall shift model may potentially reduce the total number of sign-outs by significantly staggering shift start times.[28]

A significantly different shift type that has been proposed is the float shift. Float shifts entail a dedicated provider assigned to care for boarding patients, allowing other providers to see a greater number of new patients (1.1 patients per hour more in one study).[29] This finding accords with data from a study of resident physicians, which has suggested that patients who are in observation status impose a greater productivity burden than other signed-out patients.[4] Although this additional shift is likely an effective means of improving the overall productivity and throughput of the ED, it creates a new attending shift that is not RVU-generating, which must be considered when analyzing overall and individual productivity.

STAFFING
Introduction and Objectives

ED provider productivity and staffing share many common principles and are at the core of departmental cost and throughput (**Table 3**). Both must be considered in decisions of hiring, workforce management, and patient care. This section provides an overview of the following considerations:

- What is the landscape of the ED provider workforce?
- What shift timings will use that staff most efficiently?
- How many providers should be hired to staff an ED?
- What provider mix may be appropriate?

Concept	Description
Table 3	
ED staffing concepts	
Concept	Description
Rostering	Describes the number and type of providers employed or contracted
Scheduling	Describes how provider shifts are allocated to meet patient demand
Day-of-week differences	Additional hours needed on Mondays or decreased hours mid week
Seasonal shifts	Changing shifts by season (eg, summer shifts in a vacation town)
Weekend reduction	Decrease shifts on weekends by expanding length
Flex up	Avoid scheduling 12-h shifts to allow flexing up to longer shifts
Fast track	Dedicate resources to focus on lower acuity patients
Provider in triage	See patients before traditional nurse triage
Call	Add provider to schedule to be ready to come in

The Emergency Department Workforce and Costs of Staffing

As of 2018, approximately 44,000 physicians and 14,000 APPs were working in US EDs. Of the physicians, 80% are trained in emergency medicine, with the remainder having backgrounds in other specialties. Providers trained in non-emergency medicine specialties are more prevalent in rural environments. In general, the provider labor force is very competitive, with the vast majority of emergency providers being employed by hospitals.[30–32]

ED staff make up approximately 75% to 80% of the ED-specific costs of running an ED, excluding separate hospital costs[33]; providers are a major portion of this cost. Emergency physician full-time equivalents (FTEs) have a national mean compensation of 300,000 to 472,000 USD per year. Compensation varies significantly by region and institution, and ED directors looking to hire or change compensation should survey regional competitive rates.[34] Data on APP compensation is more limited, although it can be expected that an APP salary will be at least 100,000 USD per year, in addition to other benefits.[35]

Understanding Patient Demand

Patient demand concepts

Patient demand is primarily measured by ED arrivals, usually recorded as the number of patients arriving at a given hour. ED census, or how many patients are in the ED at one time, is useful to measure workload, identifying peak load and crisis situations, and managing bed capacity (**Table 4**). Most arrival curves follow a "whale curve" (**Fig. 1**), which is used in the case study in this article, along with the corresponding census. Note that peak ED census tends to occur a few hours after the period of peak ED arrivals, and how the curve is generally flatter. Administrators must understand their own demand curves to rationalize and monitor their staffing strategy.

Patient demand and variability

Some of the greatest challenges to ED staffing are the multiple dimensions by which ED patient demand can vary, including the following.

- The 24-hour ED cycle. As depicted in **Fig. 1**, more patients typically arrive during the day than during the night (particularly 10 AM to 10 PM). Peak ED census often continues for hours even after patient arrivals begins to decrease.[36]

Table 4	
Patient demand concepts	
Concept	**Description**
ED census	How many patients are in the ED at one time
ED arrivals	How many patients arrive in a given time interval (usually by hour)
EMS arrivals	Number of EMS arrivals in a given time interval (typically have more complex care needs)
Arrivals by ESI	Number of arrivals in a given time interval stratified by emergency severity index (allows for resource allocation)
Vertical patients	Ambulatory patients, who typically demand fewer resources

- *Day-of-week variability.* There is a fairly predictable variation by day-of-week in patient visits (**Fig. 2**). Monday is typically the busiest day of the week.[37] Even within the same day of the week, a director can expect as much as 30% to 40% variation in ED patient volume.
- *Seasonal variability.* There are well-documented seasonal differences in ED volume related to certain common diseases, for example, the winter flu and viral illness season.[38] Some centers also exist in regions with major seasonal population differences, for example, a summer resort town.

It is no small challenge to account for these different factors. A reasonable rule of thumb is to measure and visualize patient arrivals per hour based on historical data and then staff provider capacity to meet patient demand up to the 70th to 80th percentile. The case study provides a closer look. With this starting point, directors can begin to account for additional dimensions of variation.

Staffing to Demand

Rostering
Multiple strategies can be used for determining the number of FTEs needed on staff.

- *Minimum single provider coverage.* Even the lowest volume EDs will have a bare minimum number of 5 FTEs on staff to provide 24/7 coverage (ie, 168 hours of coverage per week) and account for provider vacation and coverage.[30,39]
- *Generic approach to estimate FTEs.* Once annual volume is greater than 18,000 to 20,000 visits, one can estimate needing approximately 2.8 FTEs of coverage per 10,000 patient visits.[40]

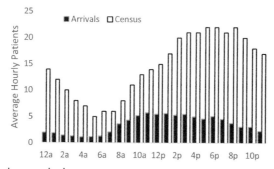

Fig. 1. Arrivals and census by hour.

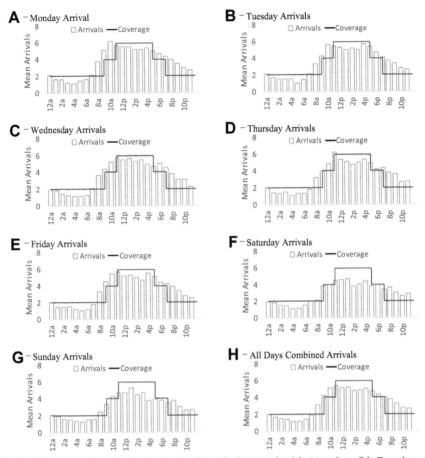

Fig. 2. Mean hourly arrivals for each day of the week; (a) Monday, (b) Tuesday, (c) Wednesday, (d) Thursday, (e) Friday, (f) Saturday, (g) Sunday, (h) All Days Combined

- *Specific approach to estimate FTEs.* Providers at different centers may have different mean productivity. Some groups may consider a physician an FTE even if fewer than 40 hours per week are spent on ED clinical work. A more sophisticated approach looks at specific parameters to make a more accurate estimate:
  1. (Annual patient visits covered per FTE) = (Mean provider patients per hour) × (clinical hours worked by FTE per week) × (nonvacation weeks worked per year by FTE)
  2. (Number FTEs required) = (Annual patient visits)/(Annual patient visits covered per FTE)
- *Hiring APPs.* Accurate estimation for APP FTEs is more challenging, because APP productivity is harder to measure given its intersection with attending physician productivity. One approach is to work backwards once a need for APP shifts is identified in the schedule, and then to hire sufficient APPs to cover the number of estimated shifts needed. This process can be beneficial when additional provider coverage is needed during certain hours, but attending coverage will be expensive and provide excess productivity.

Scheduling

Once sufficient providers are on staff, the challenge is allocating their clinical capacity to patient demand.

Shift length In general, 8- to 10-hour shifts provide more ability to flex up and account for variability and complexity. Smaller centers may not be able to avoid 12-hour shifts, to allow for sufficient days off. Longer shifts can also be used at undesirable times (eg, weekends, nights, holidays, etc) to decrease how often providers must work during those periods of time.

Set base single-provider coverage The most common strategies involve shifts starting at 0700, 1500, and 2300 for 8-hour shifts or 0700 and 1900 for 12-hour shifts. This is the framework upon which additional shifts will be laid.

Graph patient demand versus provider capacity Provider capacity is usually graphed based on flat productivity. Areas where provider capacity is greater than patient arrivals represent excess capacity. Areas where patient demand is higher represent periods when the department may be understaffed (**Fig. 3**).

Allocate additional providers based on demand Once single coverage is deemed inadequate, static modeling should be used to determine where to add additional coverage. See Patient Demand and Variability as well as the Case Study elsewhere in this article. Adding an APP is a more cost-effective step for a small excess of demand, with more complicated mixes of physicians and APPs required for larger units of unmet demand.

Complex Scheduling

- *Fast track.* Fast track is a form of split flow that diverts low-acuity patients to be seen by dedicated providers, typically in a dedicated space. It is usually staffed by 1 provider, with coverage by APPs used to meet additional demand. Studies have estimated that an APP will see approximately 2.2 patients per hour in a fast track setting.[5] Although the RVU per patient of these patients tends to be low, the support for flow can significantly reduce the likelihood of running out of beds.

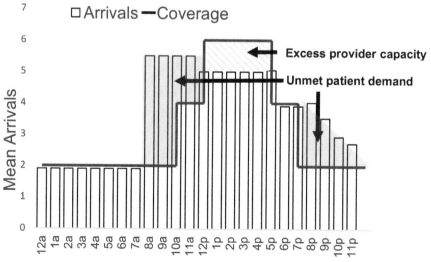

Fig. 3. Patient demand versus provider capacity.

- *Provider-in-triage (PIT)*. A PIT model creates complicated challenges for staffing, because it is difficult to measure how much patient demand is covered by this provider. There is limited evidence that a senior PIT is more effective than staffing an APP or resident in decreasing wait times and length of stay; however, the cost of this factor must be considered when assessing this intervention.[41] A general approach would be to staff the PIT area during times that the waiting room tends to be most full. Alternatively, a phased approach can be considered, where the PIT model is not activated until ED beds are full (as measured by ED census). The PIT model can significantly improve quality measures, such as arrival to provider times, and start diagnostic testing earlier, which decreased bottlenecks.
- *Dynamic solutions—Queuing theory, simulation, and computer modeling*. Matching provider capacity to patient demand has limits. In complex systems with split flow, multiple zones of patient care, triage providers, and rate-limiting factors outside of ED control, computer simulation may be required to determine where additional provider time will best improve patient throughput.

Staffing Limitations

- *Patient demand varies*. Staffing plans assume a predictable pattern of patient arrivals and complexity. There are meaningful trends, but they will not predict your ED census tomorrow. Design a phased plan for surge and crises.
- *Provider productivity varies*. Not all providers have the same speed and skill. Even the same provider may differ in performance from one day to the next when overworked, stressed, or purely by chance.
- *Hourly provider productivity is not flat*. Standard demand–capacity modeling assumes a constant patients per hour, when it has been shown that physician productivity decreases during the course of a shift (**Fig. 4**).[2]
- *Staffing for the mean*. A department staffed for the mean volume will be understaffed and in crisis 50% of the time, which can lead to issues with patient safety and burnout. A department that is always staffed for the busiest days on record will be financially unsustainable. The right answer is likely in between, and many departments staff for the 75%ile of patient arrivals.
- *The human element of staffing*. Staffing involves people who have needs and preferences that go beyond the throughput of the department.

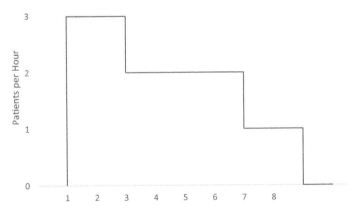

Fig. 4. Staircase model of provider productivity.

○ Nights and weekends may be intentionally understaffed if providers value minimizing the number of these shifts. Consider paying a higher rate for these shifts (subtracted from other shifts to stay cost neutral).
○ Older providers may have greater challenges working overnights. A one-size-fits-all model for scheduling may not support individual provider needs.
○ Centers with regular high acuity at night may want to avoid single coverage, even if on average night providers will not work to capacity.

ED leaders must be aware of these considerations to make the department a more desirable place to work.

CASE STUDY

You are a new ED director and have taken on the responsibility to staff and manage the productivity of your department that sees an average of 80 visits per day (about 30,000 per year). You currently staff 40 physician-hours per day, with all days of the week having the same shifts. This costs roughly $2 million per year. After interviewing the staff on where they see issues and opportunities, you note the following concerns.

- Mondays are brutal on staff, and patients often complain about long wait times.
- Night shifts often start with many patients in the waiting room.
- Physicians are burning out and scheduling is a challenge when anyone goes on vacation.
- Resentment is growing owing to variability in perceived physician effort.

You decide to take a data-driven approach by working through the steps of understanding patient demand, staffing to that demand, rostering, scheduling, and measuring variability in productivity. Data in the hospital electronic medical record system logs information for each patient, including arrival time, provider name, provider time, disposition, disposition time, and depart time.

Understanding Patient Demand

To understand patient demand, you visualize demand by hour of day, day of week, month of year, and between years, as shown in **Fig. 5**. This modeling demonstrates that Mondays have about 10% more patients per day than the other days of the week, summer and winter tend to have higher demand than average, and that year over year demand is increasing. Demand varies significantly across the day, and follows a whale curve. More research finds that the shift map has not changed since the beginning of 2017, meaning the average patients per hour has increased from 1.9 to 2.1 (13% increase). Additional analysis finds that summer Mondays in 2019 averaged 92 patients (2.3 patients per hour), with several extreme days having more than 100 patients.

The current shifts are 0700 to 1500, 0900 to 1900, 1100 to 2100, 1500 to 2300, and 2300 to 0700. **Fig. 2** shows these shifts plotted alongside the mean patient arrivals by day of week, assuming 2.0 patients per hour capacity for every hour of every shift. The productivity target should be a true average of productivity, not how hard your providers are working at peak load, or your department will feel understaffed one-half of the time (providers cannot sustainably operate above peak load). Note how in **Fig. 2**A, patient demand is not met at 9 PM, 10 PM, and 11 PM , which suggest significant queueing for the night shift.

Using the data collected, you form a table of operational metrics (**Table 5**), including mean daily arrivals (by day of week) and physician hours scheduled. Dividing arrivals by

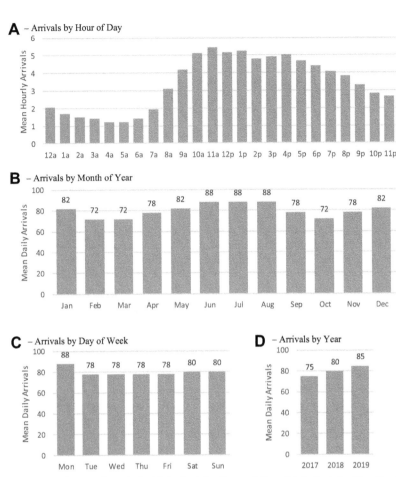

Fig. 5. Mean daily arrival analysis; (a) Arrivals by Hour of Day, (b) Arrivals by Month of Year, (c) Arrivals by Day of Week, (d) Arrivals by Year

physician hours gives the effective patients per hour productivity of the physicians working on that day of the week. This is one estimate of your provider workload and adequacy of staffing. In addition, you record *median* arrival-to-provider, provider-to-disposition (PtD) times, and the *mean* rates of left before being seen.[42] PtD can be further divided into admitted and discharged patients (PtD-A and PtD-D). These metrics are useful for determining when providers have been stretched beyond peak capacity and when the ED is reaching a peak load crisis. Recording disposition to departure from the ED for admitted patients (DtD-A) can identify when the system is experiencing dysfunction owing to processes outside the ED (such as an inpatient bed crisis).

These measures can be tracked by month to assess the change in performance after the staffing adjustments are made. Finally, provider satisfaction should be considered as changes are made.

Staffing to Demand

Based on these findings and your department benchmark of 2.0 patients per hour, you divide the average number of patient arrivals each day in the table by 2.0. You determine that Mondays should have 44 hours of coverage, and the other days of the week

Table 5
Performance measures by day of week

DOW	Arrivals	Patients per Hour	Arrival-to-Provider Time (Min)	PtD-D (Min)	PtD-A (Min)	DtD-A (Min)	LOS (Min)	LWBS (%)
Mon	88	2.2	28	126	252	175	305	5.1
Tue	78	2.0	12	72	144	180	265	2.4
Wed	78	2.0	13	78	156	175	270	2.6
Thu	78	2.0	14	81	162	195	260	2.5
Fri	78	2.0	13	75	150	190	265	2.4
Sat	80	2.0	15	90	180	184	275	2.6
Sun	80	2.0	16	105	210	191	270	2.5

should have 40 hours of coverage. You assess the periods of excess patient demand on Mondays and adjust your schedule as shown in **Table 6**.

You plot the patient demand versus the original and new patient capacity in **Fig. 6**A, B, respectively. However, you recall that provider productivity is nonlinear, with the first hour of each shift seeing significantly more patients than a normal hour, and the last hour of each shift seeing significantly fewer. To incorporate this important staffing concept without creating unrealistic complexity, you decide to increase the first hour's assumed productivity to 3 patients per hour, and decrease the last hour to half productivity. The before and after nonlinear Mondays are shown in **Fig. 6**C, D, respectively, with the staircase assumptions.

Expanding Monday coverage and level-loading capacity to demand, especially in the evening, should improve the difficulty of Mondays, and decrease the number of patients in the waiting room before the night shift. Short shifts were chosen to allow for flexing up. Tracking key performance indicators and surveying providers will help you to understand if the new staffing produces both measurable and perceived improvement.

Rostering and Scheduling

To understand the need for expanding the roster, you pull the hours worked by week for each physician. Although the average hours worked per week is 36, you find that several physicians are working more than 40 hours per week. In addition, not only did these physicians work a large number of hours, they frequently worked consecutive shifts starting at significantly different times of the day. Both the hours and variability in shift time contributed to burnout, and kept the ED as crisis-level work. To add 4 additional hours per week and keep all providers at 36 hours per week, you decide to hire an additional FTE. You also implement restrictions on scheduling, such that no shift can start more than 2 hours earlier than the previous day's shift.

Table 6
Revised shift structure

Day of Week \ Shift Number	1	2	3	4	5
Mon	0700–1500	0900–1700	1100–2100	1500–2300	2100–0700
Tue-Sun	0700–1500	0900–1600	1200–2000	1400–2200	2200-0700

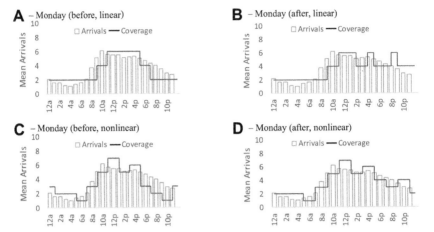

Fig. 6. Mondays before and after shift adjustment; (a) Monday (before, linear), (b) Monday (after, linear), (c) Monday (before, nonlinear), (d) Monday (after, nonlinear)

Recognizing that the solution increased costs for the ED, you research developing an APP program, developing a scribe program, and implementing lean process improvements. Your long-term goal is to have one-half of the ED staffed by APPs, increase the overall number of hours worked, and decrease the overall total staffing cost. Quarterly reviews of productivity support an incentive program based on RVUs generated. You continuously track your operational data and use it to support staffing updates.

SUMMARY

Higher productivity and staffing to demand are fundamental goals of ED operations. However, a single-minded drive to greater productivity can risk tradeoffs, including a lower quality of care, lower patient and provider satisfaction, and compromised handoffs. It is critical for ED leaders to simultaneously manage and balance productivity, quality, and timeliness of care, with both provider and patient experience. This process is ongoing and requires significant investments of time in listening to the concerns of staff, acquiring accurate data, and coordinating with other departments.

Part of the ED management journey is acknowledging that much of the improvement opportunities lie not just in enhancing people, processes, and technology, but also in enhancing the interfaces with other departments. Much of this involves situational awareness, such as knowing when other departments change shifts (eg, nursing), aligning incentives (eg, inpatient physicians), ensuring resource availability (eg, radiology), and keeping open lines of communication with other leaders.

DISCLOSURE

The authors have nothing to disclose.

REFERENCES

1. Kairouz VF, Raad D, Fudyma J, et al. Assessment of faculty productivity in academic departments of medicine in the United States: a national survey. BMC Med Educ 2014;14:205.

2. Joseph JW, Davis S, Wilker EH, et al. Modelling attending physician productivity in the emergency department: a multicentre study. Emerg Med J 2018;35(5): 317–22.

3. Joseph JW, Henning DJ, Strouse CS, et al. Modeling Hourly resident productivity in the emergency department. Ann Emerg Med 2017;70(2):185–90.e6.

4. Joseph JW, Stenson BA, Dubosh NM, et al. The effect of signed-out emergency department patients on resident productivity. J Emerg Med 2018;55(2):244–51.

5. Jeanmonod R, Delcollo J, Jeanmonod D, et al. Comparison of resident and mid-level provider productivity and patient satisfaction in an emergency department fast track. Emerg Med J 2013;30(1):e12.

6. Hamden K, Jeanmonod D, Gualtieri D, et al. Comparison of resident and mid-level provider productivity in a high-acuity emergency department setting. Emerg Med J 2014;31(3):216–9.

7. Dowd MD, Tarantino C, Barnett TM, et al. Resident efficiency in a pediatric emergency department. Acad Emerg Med 2005;12(12):1240–4.

8. Henning DJ, McGillicuddy DC, Sanchez LD. Evaluating the effect of emergency residency training on productivity in the emergency department. J Emerg Med 2013;45(3):414–8.

9. Chakravarthy B, Posadas E, Ibrahim D, et al. Increasing off-service resident productivity while on their emergency department rotation using shift cards. J Emerg Med 2015;48(4):499–505.

10. Brennan DF, Silvestri S, Sun JY, et al. Progression of emergency medicine resident productivity. Acad Emerg Med 2007;14(9):790–4.

11. Deveau JP, Lorenz JE, Hughes MJ. Emergency medicine resident work productivity and procedural accomplishment. J Am Osteopath Assoc 2003;103(6): 291–6.

12. Thibodeau LG, Geary SP, Werter C. An evaluation of resident work profiles, attending-resident teaching interactions, and the effect of variations in emergency department volume on each. Acad Emerg Med 2010;17(Suppl 2):S62–6.

13. Joseph JW, Chiu DT, Wong ML, et al. Experience within the emergency department and improved productivity for first-year residents in emergency medicine and other specialties. West J Emerg Med 2018;19(1):128–33.

14. Clinkscales JD, Fesmire FM, Hennings JR, et al. The effect of emergency medicine residents on clinical efficiency and staffing requirements. Acad Emerg Med 2016;23(1):78–82.

15. Bhat R, Dubin J, Maloy K. Impact of learners on emergency medicine attending physician productivity. West J Emerg Med 2014;15(1):41–4.

16. Chan L, Kass LE. Impact of medical student preceptorship on ED patient throughput time. Am J Emerg Med 1999;17(1):41–3.

17. Cobb T, Jeanmonod D, Jeanmonod R. The impact of working with medical students on resident productivity in the emergency department. West J Emerg Med 2013;14(6):585–9.

18. Berger TJ, Ander DS, Terrell ML, et al. The impact of the demand for clinical productivity on student teaching in academic emergency departments. Acad Emerg Med 2004;11(12):1364–7.

19. Begaz T, Decker MC, Treat R, et al. No relationship between measures of clinical efficiency and teaching effectiveness for emergency medicine faculty. Emerg Med J 2011;28(1):37–9.

20. Kelly SP, Shapiro N, Woodruff M, et al. The effects of clinical workload on teaching in the emergency department. Acad Emerg Med 2007;14(6):526–31.

21. Hemphill RR, Heavrin BS, Lesnick J, et al. Those who can, do and they teach too: faculty clinical productivity and teaching. West J Emerg Med 2011;12(2):254–7.

22. Arya R, Salovich DM, Ohman-Strickland P, et al. Impact of scribes on performance indicators in the emergency department. Acad Emerg Med 2010;17(5): 490–4.

23. Hess JJ, Wallenstein J, Ackerman JD, et al. Scribe Impacts on Provider Experience, Operations, and Teaching in an Academic Emergency Medicine Practice. West J Emerg Med 2015;16(5):602–10.

24. Cabilan CJ, Eley RM. Review article: potential of medical scribes to allay the burden of documentation and enhance efficiency in Australian emergency departments. Emerg Med Australas 2015;27(6):507–11.

25. Thomas H Jr, Schwartz E, Whitehead DC. Eight- versus 12-hour shifts: implications for emergency physicians. Ann Emerg Med 1994;23(5):1096–100.

26. Jeanmonod R, Jeanmonod D, Ngiam R. Resident productivity: does shift length matter? Am J Emerg Med 2008;26(7):789–91.

27. Jeanmonod RK, Brook C, Winther M, et al. Dedicated shift wrap-up time does not improve resident sign-out volume or efficiency. West J Emerg Med 2010; 11(1):35–9.

28. Yoshida H, Rutman LE, Chen J, et al. Waterfalls and handoffs: a novel physician staffing model to decrease handoffs in a pediatric emergency department. Ann Emerg Med 2019;73(3):248–54.

29. Nasim MU, Mistry C, Harwood R, et al. An attending physician float shift for the improvement of physician productivity in a crowded emergency department. World J Emerg Med 2013;4(1):10–4.

30. Moorhead JC, Gallery ME, Hirshkorn C, et al. A study of the workforce in emergency medicine: 1999. Ann Emerg Med 2002;40(1):3–15.

31. Ginde AA, Sullivan AF, Camargo CA Jr. National study of the emergency physician workforce, 2008. Ann Emerg Med 2009;54(3):349–59.

32. Hall MK, Burns K, Carius M, et al. State of the national emergency department workforce: who provides care where? Ann Emerg Med 2018;72(3):302–7.

33. Bamezai A, Melnick G, Nawathe A. The cost of an emergency department visit and its relationship to emergency department volume. Ann Emerg Med 2005; 45(5):483–90.

34. 2018-2019 Compensation Report for Emergency Physicians - ACEP Now. ACEP Now. Available at: https://www.acepnow.com/article/2018-2019-compensation-report-for-emergency-physicians/. Accessed November 1, 2019.

35. Physician-Assistant Salary." Best Healthcare Jobs, U.S. News and World Report. Available at: https://money.usnews.com/careers/best-jobs/physician-assistant/salary. Accessed February 25, 2020.

36. Welch SJ, Jones SS, Allen T. Mapping the 24-hour emergency department cycle to improve patient flow. Jt Comm J Qual Patient Saf 2007;33(5):247–55.

37. Asplin BR, Flottemesch TJ, Gordon BD. Developing models for patient flow and daily surge capacity research. Acad Emerg Med 2006;13(11):1109–13.

38. Shaw KN, Lavelle JM. VESAS: a solution to seasonal fluctuations in emergency department census. Ann Emerg Med 1998;32(6):698–702.

39. van de Leuv JH. Physician staffing. Management of Emergency Services 1987; 2:35.

40. Holley JE, Kellermann AL, Andrulis DP. Physician staffing in the emergency departments of public teaching hospitals: a national survey. Ann Emerg Med 1992;21(1):53–7.

41. Abdulwahid MA, Booth A, Kuczawski M, et al. The impact of senior doctor assessment at triage on emergency department performance measures: systematic review and meta-analysis of comparative studies. Emerg Med J 2016;33(7): 504–13.
42. Wiler JL, Welch S, Pines J, et al. Emergency department performance measures updates: proceedings of the 2014 emergency department benchmarking alliance consensus summit. Acad Emerg Med 2015;22(5):542–53.

Patient Assignment Models in the Emergency Department

Nicole R. Hodgson, MD*, Stephen J. Traub, MD

KEYWORDS

- Rotational patient assignment • Provider in triage • Fast track
- Emergency department operations • Physician assignment

KEY POINTS

- Patient assignment systems are front-end operational tactics that can improve emergency department length of stay, rate of patients leaving without being seen, patient satisfaction, and resident education.
- There are multiple variations of patient assignment systems, including provider-in-triage/team triage, fast-tracks/vertical pathways, and rotational patient assignment.
- The patient assignment component of both provider-in-triage/team triage and fast-tracks/vertical pathways is likely to generate the greatest operational improvements in emergency departments with large numbers of lower-acuity patients.
- The patient assignment component of rotational patient assignment is likely to generate the greatest operational improvements in emergency departments in which there is neither guidance nor obvious incentives (such as financial) to encourage physicians to acquire ("pick up") patients.

INTRODUCTION

As emergency departments (EDs) around the world struggle to accommodate ever-growing numbers of patients,[1] novel workflow solutions are needed. This innovation is critical, because the traditional approach to crowding, building a larger ED, does not always reduce crowding.[2] Workflow smoothing often matters more than physical layout. Some EDs have experimented with patient assignment systems, where early assignment of patients to specific treatment teams has been found to improve patients' length of stay,[3] rates of leaving without being seen,[3,4] the quality of resident education,[5,6] and patient satisfaction.[3,4] In this article, the authors discuss the theory behind patient assignment systems and review variations and the potential benefits of different patient assignment strategies found in current literature.

Department of Emergency Medicine, Mayo Clinic Arizona, Mayo Clinic Hospital, 5777 East Mayo Boulevard, Phoenix, AZ 85054, USA
* Corresponding author.
E-mail address: Hodgson.nicole@mayo.edu

Emerg Med Clin N Am 38 (2020) 607–615
https://doi.org/10.1016/j.emc.2020.03.003
0733-8627/20/© 2020 Elsevier Inc. All rights reserved.

emed.theclinics.com

THEORY OF EMERGENCY DEPARTMENT PATIENT ASSIGNMENT SYSTEMS

Traditional queue management theory teaches that pooling identical customers into 1 centralized pool, attended by multiple similar servers, increases efficiency by decreasing the amount of time a customer waits.[7] Many EDs use a "pooled" workflow whereby any emergency physician can treat any patient. However, unlike the "customers" that queue management addresses, patients are not identical, nor are physicians. Patients with unique medical backgrounds present with a broad range of chief complaints and needs. Physicians also appear to have inherent traits that affect their workflow, including risk-aversion[8] and fear of malpractice.[9] These inherent traits may help to explain the observation that many clinicians can be stereotyped as having a "high" or "low" resource utilization profile.[10] These and other aspects of emergency medicine workflow suggest that queuing theory may require modification when assessing some aspects of ED operations.

Most EDs rely on physicians assigning themselves to waiting patients, voluntarily taking on additional work. However, physicians may not always act as perfect workers, because burnout, fatigue, and other factors can lead to behaviors that decrease efficiency. Physicians may "foot-drag," delaying disposition of assigned patients, in order to increase their apparent workload when patients are assigned by a monitoring nurse manager.[11] Placing ED physicians in close physical proximity to one another and allowing them to self-assign patients appear to decrease this foot-dragging behavior, possibly because of peer pressure; however, "social loafing," whereby individual workers decrease their effort in a group setting, may come into play as physicians wait to see whether other physicians self-assign to less-desirable patients.[12] This process is also referred to as "cherry-picking" and has been described in resident physicians.[13]

An automated system of patient assignment may decrease foot-dragging and social loafing by making these tendencies, in effect, counterproductive. If an individual ED physician is given a queue of his or her own patients without regard for workload, overall length of stay for patients decreases.[3,14] One possible reason is that pooled queues may not be optimal for "strategic servers" such as physicians, who have the ability to adjust the amount of time they spend on tasks and the order in which they take on duties.[14] In 1 example, patients were assigned to physicians at the time of triage. Physicians were expected to disposition their patients before shift completion, thereby incentivizing more efficient practice because these physicians were salaried and not compensated for additional work time. The assignment system appeared to counteract what had been a consistent slowing previously noted near the end of shifts, resulting in improvements in length of stay.[14]

Work prioritization also bears mention. ED physicians have multiple simultaneous tasks competing for their attention and must balance attention to old patients with seeing new patients. Intuitively, salaried compensation models would seem to favor the first behavior, whereas productivity-based models would favor the second. Patient assignment models may fare differently based on the compensation scheme at a facility, with rotational patient assignment models likely having their greatest benefit in those departments with less incentive to acquire new patients.

CATEGORIES OF PATIENT ASSIGNMENT SYSTEMS

Several versions of patient assignment systems exist in the literature, and these interventions fall into 3 broad categories. For two (provider in triage/team triage and fast-track/vertical pathways), patient assignment is a relatively minor component of the strategy; for one (rotational patient assignment), it is the central component.

PATIENT ASSIGNMENT TO TRIAGE TEAMS

A single provider or multidisciplinary team may be used in place of a nurse in triage.[15] Earlier contact between physician and patient should theoretically lead to a shorter length of stay for that patient, because needed interventions can be initiated earlier. The use of a specific style of provider varies; attending physicians,[16] physician assistants,[17] and residents[18] have all been shown to provide potential benefits in this role.

One multidisciplinary triage team, called the Supplemental Triage And Rapid Treatment (START), improved length of stay for both discharged and admitted patients.[17] In this approach, an attending physician assessed the patient in the triage area, identified patients suitable for the START program, and placed initial orders. A midlevel provider working side by side with this physician followed the patient's care plan to completion. Although the ED already used a fast-track area, this new team successfully dispositioned approximately 20% of patients from triage, and this percentage increased to 29% in the 3-year follow-up assessment.[19] This model relies on the triage physician to identify patients suitable for the pathway, self-assigning patients to their care team and removing patients from the main ED waiting room pool. Similar programs at other hospitals resulted in 34.8%[20] and 48.9%[21] of patients being discharged from the triage area without being assigned to physicians in the main ED.

Empowering a triage team to disposition patients may work well in hospital systems seeing large numbers of lower-acuity patients. However, there are limitations to this method, particularly when compared with other forms of patient assignment.

First, this approach relies entirely on the motivation of the treating triage team. Many of the benefits of using a provider in triage stem from early dispositions and self-assignment of less complex patients from the waiting room pool. A hospital where triage teams initiate workup and transfer care to the main ED may not achieve the same benefits as those that focus on treating patients primarily for early dispositions. In 1 facility in which an additional shift for a physician in triage led to an overall improvement in length of stay,[22] secondary analysis of the data revealed that patients dispositioned by the triage physician had a dramatically decreased length of stay, whereas patients who had triage orders placed and their care transferred to another physician in the main ED had an increased length of stay. One possible explanation is that 55% of these patients had additional tests ordered by the second physician. Institutions with greater provider variability may benefit from selection of another model of patient assignment instead of using a provider in triage.

Second, most publications report benefits when adding a provider shift to cover the triage area, begging the question of whether adding a provider shift to the main ED instead may have brought about similar or even superior results. In 1 series of experiments, when a provider was added to triage, there was an improvement in throughput that disappeared if that provider was instead repurposed from fast track.[23,24] In a pediatric ED with a preexisting fast track, the reallocation of existing staff to place a provider in triage resulted in an improvement in length of stay for patients categorized as "urgent" or "nonurgent" but prolonged length of stay for "emergent" patients[25]; this is a trade-off that must be considered at the individual hospital level.

Finally, patient satisfaction may suffer. Although some studies report improvement in patient satisfaction scores with the use of a provider in triage,[26] others have found the opposite.[27]

PATIENT ASSIGNMENT TO FAST-TRACK AND VERTICAL PATHWAYS

Another model in which patient assignment plays a role is in the streaming of patients into different areas of the ED, staffed by separate providers, based on their initial presentation. This most common version of this model is a "fast-track."

In EDs using a "fast track," patients triaged as lower acuity or predicted to require limited resources are assigned to a specific area of the department. Physicians[28,29] or midlevel providers[30,31] then staff this area in partnership with an ED nurse or technician. Fast tracks can be effective in decreasing patient wait time[28] and length of stay[29,31] while improving patient satisfaction.[31] A variety of EDs have achieved success using a fast track, including trauma-only departments[28] and those at pediatric hospitals.[29]

Fast-track areas may improve throughput and resource utilization by modifying providers' approach toward patients. One pediatric study identified strict criteria (well-appearing children ages 2 months to 10 years with no history of immunocompromise or chronic conditions, presenting with a chief complaint of fever, vomiting, diarrhea, or decreased oral intake) to indicate suitability for a fast track. At times when the fast track was closed, these patients would be treated in the main ED. Assignment to the fast track resulted in improved length of stay as well as decreased rates of test utilization, admission, and intravenous fluid administration. Follow-up calls revealed that there were no statistically significant rates of self-reported improvement, unscheduled follow-up visits, and patient satisfaction between the groups treated in the fast track or the ED.[29] This finding suggests that some aspect of the fast-track environment encouraged treating physicians to decrease their own resource utilization without compromising clinical quality, possibly because of increased efficiency pressures or a "bias toward wellness." The study investigators also posit that the fast-track environment may have had a calming effect on the children when compared with the ED, making them less fussy and therefore more well appearing. Whether such an effect is generalizable to adult EDs remains to be seen.

"Vertical pathways," like fast tracks, assign ambulatory patients to specific ED providers in a dedicated area; the hallmark of vertical pathways, as the name suggests, is that patients are not placed horizontally onto stretchers. Whereas fast tracks tend to focus on Emergency Severity Index (ESI) 4/5 patients, vertical streaming often targets ambulatory ESI 3s. In 1 study, an ED with a preexisting fast track found added benefits when converting typical patient rooms to vertical zones.[32]

Advanced use of the fast-track/vertical pathway model includes using discrete event simulation to determine the number of fast-track beds to convert to "flexible" beds that could be preferentially given to high-acuity patients unless the main ED was not at capacity.[33]

ROTATIONAL PATIENT ASSIGNMENT

The patient assignment aspects of provider in triage/team triage and fast-track/vertical pathway models may work best for EDs managing large numbers of low-acuity patients. However, EDs with higher acuity may benefit from other models. Rotational patient assignment, whereby patients are algorithmically assigned to physicians working in the main ED, has proven successful in several settings, including those with high-acuity patients.

In 1 example of a rotational patient assignment system,[3] patients are automatically and algorithmically assigned to an ED physician upon registration via a computer program integrated with the medical record. Physicians receive 4 sequential patients at the beginning of their shift and are then placed into a rotational queue with other physicians who are on shift. Physicians are removed from the queue when they have received a predetermined maximum number of patients for the shift or 2 hours before their shift is scheduled to end (whichever comes first) to allow physicians to appropriately disposition their patients before leaving. Patients are triaged and placed into rooms according to acuity, irrespective of physician assignment, and can be placed into any physical location within the ED.

The assignment program does not take patient acuity into account. Physicians are empowered and encouraged to trade with one another if an unsafe situation is encountered (2 simultaneous cardiac arrests assigned to 1 physician, for example). Practically, however, such trading is rare. Physician shifts are staggered throughout the day at intervals to optimally align provider availability with typical departmental patient arrival curves. If too many patients arrive for the designated physician shifts, an on-call provider is activated to help manage the load, but this (like patient trading) is a rare occurrence.

Changing from a typical physician self-assignment model to the above-described rotational patient assignment system was associated with significant operational improvements, including decreases in median length of stay (11%), arrival to provider evaluation (44%), rate of left without being seen (51%), and complaints (40%). Every physician in the group had a lower length of stay after the intervention, including those who were previously the fastest. Anecdotally, physicians reported improved satisfaction with the rotational system, which they describe as "brutally fair." Nurses also report benefits, because they immediately know which physician to approach with abnormal electrocardiograms, requests for pain medications, or other concerns. This model has delivered sustained operational improvements with only minor changes to the system over recent years.[34]

One study that compared the above model to the physician in triage noted no statistically significant difference in length of stay between the 2 models,[16] but elected to use rotational patient assignment because of physician and nursing preference and a subjective belief that rotational patient assignment was a superior workflow.

One difficult constraint in this model is lack of space as it relates to the timing of patient assignment. If a computerized system assigns patients to physicians at the time of arrival, ED boarding and wait times for emergency bed availability can have an outsized impact on the ability of physicians to see their assigned patients. In periods of peak volume, physicians may be assigned to multiple patients in the waiting room with no dedicated space to evaluate them. One solution would be to switch the time of assignment from patient arrival to assignment to a physical bed, although this would likely result in the loss of several efficiencies. In an assignment-on-arrival system, physicians generally monitor their patients in the waiting room, review electronic records, order initial tests, and alert the charge nurse to abnormal vitals or concerning histories that may not have been detected in triage. Physicians may walk to the waiting room to meet their patients during triage or use set-aside areas adjacent to the waiting room to perform a brief initial history or physical examination. Literature supports the decision to keep assignment at the time of patient arrival, because wait time[35] and length of stay[14,35] are both improved when patients are assigned at the time of arrival compared with the time of bedding.

In a second example, patients were assigned to teams consisting of an ED physician, 2 ED nurses, and an ED technician.[4] The assignment was made after the initial nursing triage screening was complete. Room assignment depended on team assignment, with specific ED rooms assigned to each ED team. New physicians received fewer patients to their teams during their first few months of employment. Physicians stopped receiving patients 4 hours before the end of their shift and could leave whenever they completed work on all assigned patients. Implementation of this system led to improved patient satisfaction, decreased wait time, and lower rates of patients leaving without being seen.

Another variation of this model takes patient acuity into account. One ED in Hong Kong split 4 doctors into 2 separate teams.[36] Patients were split into "emergent/urgent" or "semiurgent/nonurgent" queues. Teams received patients from both queues on a rotational basis.

Several factors differed in this version of rotational patient assignment compared with those mentioned above. A senior physician who was screening incoming patients would reassign patients if wait times began to differ more than 30 minutes between the 2 teams and would begin to see patients primarily if the wait time became more than 1 hour. Because 2 physicians worked within each team and did not individually receive patient loads, this system relied much more on peer pressure and inherent physician dedication to efficiency than the above-described individual assignment systems. The study did not report several crucial operational metrics (such as length of stay) but did find a decrease in the primary outcome of patient wait time.

Rotational patient assignment has been compared with acuity-based split-flow patient streaming.[37] In the first of 2 EDs within the same Taiwanese health care system, 1 physician treated all urgent cases (designated "resuscitation" or "emergency" on arrival to triage), and an additional 2 physicians treated all other patients. In the second ED, a computerized system assigned patients in rotational fashion to the 3 physicians on shift. When compared with the split-flow department, the rotational patient assignment department demonstrated a 0.4-hour increase in length of stay for discharged patients and a 1.6-hour decrease in length of stay for patients admitted to the intensive care unit. Physicians working in the split-flow department ordered fewer laboratory tests but did not differ on rates of computed tomographic scans when compared with the physicians in the rotational assignment model. There are limitations in this study, because different physicians staffed the 2 EDs, and operational differences at each institution may have influenced results.

Academic training programs employing resident physicians have also reported success with rotational patient assignment systems. Not only do such systems benefit patients, improving length of stay[5] and patient satisfaction,[38] but they also benefit residents as well. Rotational patient assignment interventions improved resident and faculty satisfaction,[5] resident perception of quality and amount of teaching,[6] and patients seen per hour by individual residents.[6] Resident assignment systems prevent cherry-picking and ensure resident exposure to a broad range of ED cases.

One study reports the feasibility of rotational team assignment incorporating multiple levels of learners paired with nursing staff.[38] The department in question created 2 teams that received patient assignments in a rotational fashion: red (third-year emergency medicine resident, rotating intern and medical student, one or 2 nurses) and blue (second- and first-year emergency medicine residents, one or 2 nurses). Perhaps unique to this model, nurses continued to receive patient assignments even if previous assignments (patients) physically remained present in their beds; this reportedly placed additional pressure on both nursing staff and physician staff to prioritize efficiency. Attending physicians did not receive patient assignments. Patient satisfaction increased significantly with this new team-based assignment, although the article did not report on critical operational outcomes.

SUMMARY

Although simple queuing theory may suggest that "pooled" models will improve efficiency, a nuanced understanding of ED operations suggests that there are important exceptions to this rule. Patient assignment systems are deviations from simple queues that may result in improved patient flow. The improvements in throughput attributable to patient assignment may be relatively small in systems such as physician in triage/team triage and fast-track/vertical pathways, or large in systems such as rotational patient assignment.

Research examining patient assignment systems is in its infancy, with few trials published in the literature. These systems, and particularly rotational patient assignment, are associated with significant improvements in departmental operations, patient satisfaction, and resident experience when applied in an academic setting. At 1 facility, these gains have proved to be durable over time.

Patient assignment systems will likely continue to evolve as ED leaders experiment with novel methods to optimize flow. Although basic patient assignment systems have been effective, future work in this area may leverage machine learning and artificial intelligence to optimize assignments.

DISCLOSURE

The authors have nothing to disclose.

REFERENCES

1. Yarmohammadian MH, Rezaei F, Haghshenas A, et al. Overcrowding in emergency departments: a review of strategies to decrease future challenges. J Res Med Sci 2017;22:23.
2. Sayah A, Lai-Becker M, Kingsley-Rocker L, et al. Emergency department expansion versus patient flow improvement: impact on patient experience of care. J Emerg Med 2016;50(2):339–48.
3. Traub SJ, Stewart CF, Didehban R, et al. Emergency department rotational patient assignment. Ann Emerg Med 2016;67(2):206–15.
4. Patel PB, Vinson DR. Team assignment system: expediting emergency department care. Ann Emerg Med 2005;46(6):499–506.
5. Hirshon JM, Kirsch TD, Mysko WK, et al. Effect of rotational patient assignment on emergency department length of stay. J Emerg Med 1996;14(6):763–8.
6. Nable J, Greenwood J, Abraham M, et al. Implementation of a team-based physician staffing model at an academic emergency department. West J Emerg Med 2014;15(6):682–6.
7. Eppen GD. Note–effects of centralization on expected costs in a multi-location newsboy problem. Management Sci 1979;25(5):498–501.
8. Pines JM, Hollander JE, Isserman JA, et al. The association between physician risk tolerance and imaging use in abdominal pain. Am J Emerg Med 2009;27(5):552–7.
9. Katz DA, Williams GC, Brown RL, et al. Emergency physicians' fear of malpractice in evaluating patients with possible acute cardiac ischemia. Ann Emerg Med 2005;46(6):525–33.
10. Hodgson NR, Saghafian S, Mi L, et al. Are testers also admitters? Comparing emergency physician resource utilization and admitting practices. Am J Emerg Med 2018;36(10):1865–9.
11. Chan DC. Teamwork and moral hazard: evidence from the emergency department. J Polit Econ 2016;124(3):734–70.
12. Latané B, Williams K, Harkins S. Many hands make light the work: the causes and consequences of social loafing. J Personality Soc Psych 1979;37(6):822–32.

13. Patterson BW, Batt RJ, Wilbanks MD, et al. Cherry picking patients: examining the interval between patient rooming and resident self-assignment. Acad Emerg Med 2016;23(6):679–84.
14. Song H, Tucker AL, Murrell KL. The diseconomies of queue pooling: an empirical investigation of emergency department length of stay. Manage Sci 2015;61(12): 3032–53.
15. Wiler JL, Gentle C, Halfpenny JM, et al. Optimizing emergency department front-end operations. Ann Emerg Med 2010;55(2). https://doi.org/10.1016/j.annemergmed.2009.05.021.
16. Traub SJ, Bartley AC, Smith VD, et al. Physician in triage versus rotational patient assignment. J Emerg Med 2016;50(5):784–90.
17. White BA, Brown DFM, Sinclair J, et al. Supplemented Triage and Rapid Treatment (START) improves performance measures in the emergency department. J Emerg Med 2012;42(3):322–8.
18. Svirsky I, Stoneking LR, Grall K, et al. Resident-initiated advanced triage effect on emergency department patient flow. J Emerg Med 2013;45(5):746–51.
19. Rogg JG, White BA, Biddinger PD, et al. A long-term analysis of physician triage screening in the emergency department. Acad Emerg Med 2013;20(4):374–80.
20. Travers JP, Lee FCY. Avoiding prolonged waiting time during busy periods in the emergency department: is there a role for the senior emergency physician in triage? Eur J Emerg Med 2006;13(6):342–8.
21. Terris J, Leman P, O'Connor N, et al. Making an IMPACT on emergency department flow: improving patient processing assisted by consultant at triage. Emerg Med J 2004;21(5):537–41.
22. Traub SJ, Wood JP, Kelley J, et al. Emergency department rapid medical assessment: overall effect and mechanistic considerations. J Emerg Med 2015;48(5): 620–7.
23. Nestler DM, Fratzke AR, Church CJ, et al. Effect of a physician assistant as triage liaison provider on patient throughput in an academic emergency department. Acad Emerg Med 2012;19:1235–41.
24. Nestler DM, Halasy MP, Fratzke AR, et al. Patient throughput benefits of triage liaison providers are lost in a resource-neutral model: a prospective trial. Acad Emerg Med 2014;21(7):794–8.
25. Li J, Caviness A, Patel B. Effect of a rapid assessment program on total length of stay in a pediatric emergency department. Pediatr Emerg Care 2011;27(4): 295–300.
26. Weston V, Jain SK, Gottlieb M, et al. Effectiveness of resident physicians as triage liaison providers in an academic emergency department. West J Emerg Med 2017;18(4):577–84.
27. Repplinger M, Ravi S, Lee A, et al. The impact of an emergency department front-end redesign on patient-reported satisfaction survey results. West J Emerg Med 2017;18(6):1068–74.
28. Cooke MW, Wilson S, Pearson S. The effect of a separate stream for minor injuries on accident and emergency department waiting times. Emerg Med J 2002;19(1): 28–30.
29. Hampers LC, Cha S, Gutglass DJ, et al. Fast track and the pediatric emergency department: resource utilization and patient outcomes. Acad Emerg Med 1999; 6(11):1153–9.
30. Wiler JL, Ozkaynak M, Bookman K, et al. Implementation of a front-end split-flow model to promote performance in an urban academic emergency department. Jt Comm J Qual Patient Saf 2016;42(6):271–80.

31. Rodi SW, Grau MV, Orsini CM. Evaluation of a fast track unit: alignment of resources and demand results in improved satisfaction and decreased length of stay for emergency department patients. Qual Manag Health Care 2006;15(3):163–70.
32. Wallingford G, Joshi N, Callagy P, et al. Introduction of a horizontal and vertical split flow model of emergency department patients as a response to overcrowding. J Emerg Nurs 2018;44(4):345–52.
33. Laker LF, Froehle CM, Lindsell CJ, et al. The flex track: flexible partitioning between low- and high-acuity areas of an emergency department. Ann Emerg Med 2014;64(6):591–603.
34. Traub SJ, Saghafian S, Bartley AC, et al. The durability of operational improvements with rotational patient assignment. Am J Emerg Med 2018;36(8):1367–71.
35. Murrell K, Offerman SR, Martinez J, et al. 138 use of an early patient-physician assignment system on emergency department arrival decreases time to physician and emergency department length of stay. Ann Emerg Med 2012;60(4):S50.
36. Lau FL, Leung KP. Waiting time in an urban accident and emergency department–a way to improve it. Emerg Med J 2008;14(5):299–303.
37. Yau FF, Tsai TC, Lin YR, et al. Can different physicians providing urgent and non-urgent treatment improve patient flow in emergency department? Am J Emerg Med 2018;36(6):993–7.
38. DeBehnke D, Decker MC. The effects of a physician-nurse patient care team on patient satisfaction in an academic ED. Am J Emerg Med 2002;20(4):267–70.

Design of the Academic Emergency Department

Kenneth D. Marshall, MD, MA[a,b],*, Bryan Imhoff, MD, MBA[a], Frank Zilm, DArch[c]

KEYWORDS

- ED design • Throughput • Flow • Crowding • Space • Planning • Architecture

KEY POINTS

- Early clinical input is essential to generating a successful emergency department design.
- Decisions made prematurely in the design process can place severe constraints on the ability to make changes later, so decisions should be made only when necessary.
- It is important to consider which operational flow model(s) will be used when determining capacity needs and selecting designs.
- Different design schemes have inherent advantages and disadvantages, and should be chosen based on goodness of fit to the institution's needs.
- Planning for atypical patient surge events should be incorporated in the design process.

There are few decisions that will have a more significant impact on the operations of an emergency service than those related to its physical design. Over the typical 10-year period in which a health care capital investment is evaluated, safe, efficient, caring services will be provided in an environment that either supports these tasks or makes them more challenging. Staff efficiency will likewise be either enhanced or diminished, and in turn, this environment will influence staff retention, burnout, and turnover.

To the clinician, participation in the planning and design process may present unfamiliar terms, concepts, and decisions. This article outlines some of the major terms, processes, and key decisions that clinical staff will experience as a participant in emergency department (ED) design. To do this, we first explain the overall planning and design process. Second, we describe in depth 2 major process steps, namely identification of required patient capacity and determination of operational flow models. Finally, we describe 3 representative design layouts and cover their strengths and weaknesses. Throughout these discussions, we highlight the importance of

[a] Department of Emergency Medicine, University of Kansas Medical Center, 3900 Rainbow Boulevard, Kansas City, KS 66160, USA; [b] Department of History and Philosophy of Medicine, University of Kansas Medical Center, 3900 Rainbow Boulevard, Kansas City, KS 66160, USA; [c] Institute for Health and Wellness Design, The University of Kansas, 315 Marvin Hall, Lawrence, Kansas, KS 66045, USA
* Corresponding author.
E-mail address: kmarshall2@kumc.edu

Emerg Med Clin N Am 38 (2020) 617–631
https://doi.org/10.1016/j.emc.2020.04.003
0733-8627/20/© 2020 Elsevier Inc. All rights reserved.

adaptability and safety as key tenets in ED design. Regarding adaptability, we cover strategies, such as identifying opportunities for future expansion and internal reassignments, that will allow the emergency service to respond to changing demands and operational approaches. Regarding safety, we cover topics including establishing appropriate security, isolation needs, and event-scenario strategies to protect staff and respond to high-risk events.

UNDERSTANDING THE PROCESS

The planning and design process typically moves through a series of approximations envisioning future needs, starting with workload and operational assumptions, and progressing into space programming, planning, and design (**Fig. 1**). As in clinical diagnosis and treatment, initial assumptions are established, tested, revised, and then actions implemented. Each ED design presents a unique set of site-related, demand, and operational conditions, making "evidence-based" methods of study and implementation more difficult than in clinical medicine. Much of the decision-making will rely on expert judgment and trust among the team members (see **Fig. 1**).

Another major difference from clinical practice is the timescale to complete projects. Planning and design can take months, and in some cases years, to complete. Ironically, many of the key design decisions are made early in the process when the least is known about the final design strategy. It is during these early stages of space programming and design that clinical staff have the most significant opportunity to influence the final design. As the process progresses, plans become more detailed, technical, and hard to modify. It is extremely difficult to change a design once construction has begun.

Critical to the early stages of the process is maintaining an open mind to exploring operational and space alternatives. This divergent thinking process is essential to identifying the most creative solution, and differs from decision making in other contexts, especially clinical medicine. In those situations, decisions are best made as soon as necessary information is available to allow progress. The risk in early stages of design is to make premature decisions that produce irreversible constraints on the project. Thus, decisions should be made only when necessary, suspending actions until they are critical to the overall progress of the project. This allows time for reflection and potential identification of new concepts. Encouraging frank, open discussions is essential.

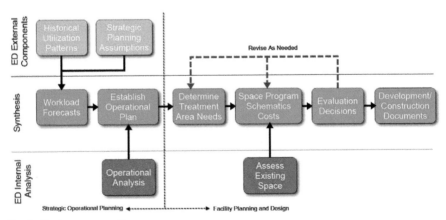

Fig. 1. Design process diagram.

Team members bring different and unique skills. Designers can be great visionaries of new ideas, but may not be skilled in quantitative techniques or clinical process needs. Clinical staff can bring important insights into care needs, but may have limited exposure to new operational and design concepts. Administration can provide strategic and financial insights but may not appreciate the impact of variability and peak demands on an emergency service. Success in the planning process is dependent on open, trusting dialogue among the team members. Site visits to other EDs early in the process can provide both valuable insights and opportunities to establish team unity.

The planning and design process typically moves through 5 phases:

- *Strategic planning:* Workload forecasts, strategic goals, identification of space elements, and basic organizational concepts are developed during this phase. Critical strategic considerations include 5-year to 10-year visit volume forecasts, throughput length of stay assumptions, anticipated operational models of care (see later in this article), and unique operational/care needs. This may be undertaken with the design architect participating or with the assistance of a planning consultant.
- *Space programming:* The insights from the strategic planning phase are used to establish key room requirements, including the number and room sizes (referred to as net square feet). The anticipated overall size of the department is also developed (departmental gross square footage [dgsf]). Target project budgets are established along with identification of major equipment purchases.
- *Schematic design:* Simple ("single line") drawings of alternative layouts of the space program with the building site are undertaken, typically relying on 2-dimensional or simple 3-dimensional drawings. Meeting budget targets are confirmed or adjusted based on these tests. A preferred concept is established during this phase.
- *Design development:* During this stage, detailed layouts of the schematic design are developed, including accurate wall and corridor dimensions, and location of headwalls, outlets, and charting areas. Full scale mock-ups of key rooms may be used to garner clinical staff input and confirmation of concepts. This is functionally the last major opportunity for clinical staff to influence the design.
- *Construction documents:* These are technical drawings and specifications primarily to solicit construction bids by outside contractors. Modifications to the ED layout or room configuration are extremely difficult to undertake, potentially risking time delays and additional professional fees.

The first 2 phases of the process require active leadership by a consistent, core clinical team. Although it is desirable to encourage participation by all interested parties, a small working group of 5 to 10 members offers an opportunity for a diverse knowledge base and the ability to meet as needed. A typical core working group should include medical, nursing, administration, facilities planning, and finance members.

Establishing a project budget during the programming and planning phase places key parameters on the project that may be difficult to change. There are 2 elements that comprise a project budget: the *construction budget* for the "brick and mortar" and the *non–construction-related costs* for equipment, site development, professional services, state reviews, and other activities. It is not uncommon for these nonconstruction budget components to equal to a quarter to a third of the project budget, particularly if major imaging equipment, such as computed tomography (CT) or MRI scanners, are in the project.

DETERMINING CAPACITY

Establishing the required number of treatment spaces for each operational component of the ED is the most significant task in the early stages of the planning and programming process. The primary challenge is identifying the impact of variability to establish peak period needs. Anticipated patient arrival patterns, treatment space needs, and length of stay must be assessed for each patient area. Dividing the problem into variables that are outside the direct control of the ED (exogenous variable) and those that are within the operational control of the service (endogenous variables) provides a logical way to manage the process.

External factors include the projected annual patient visit volume (ideally at least 5 years into the future), the demographics of the patient population and resulting treatment needs, the mix of admitted patients, and the impact of federal and local health care policies. Rather than lock into a single assumption regarding these complex issues, it is common to establish scenarios that forecast 2 or 3 potential combinations of factors. Capacity and design solutions should be evaluated against these alternative scenarios to determine the ability to meet the projected needs.

Current management concepts of LEAN[1] and Goldratt's Theory of Constraints[2] focus on identifying elements of a complex system that are impeding flow and "production." Applying this perspective to ED planning, the focus should be on arrivals and service patterns during peak periods of demand. If a department possesses enough treatment capacity to accommodate these peak periods, then meeting demand during nonpeak periods will require down-staffing to demand. At nonpeak times, space will not be the constraining variable on patient flow.

Peak period capacity can be estimated as the product of the hourly arrival rates and length of stay. This demand is then divided into the estimated available time for an appropriate treatment space, which is a function of the time (typically 1 hour) and the achievable occupancy percentage.

Treatment room needs =

$$\frac{\text{peak arrivals per hour X treatment room length of stay (minutes)}}{\text{Treatment room capacity (60 minutes * occupancy \%)}}$$

At least 3 data points should be used to adjust the annual visit forecast into peak hour demand.

1. Seasonality. Five years, or more, of historical data should be reviewed to determine if there are consistent seasonal peaks in demand. An adjustment index should be developed to incorporate identified peak seasonal demand.
2. Day of week variations. Currently many emergency services experience a Monday spike in demand for adult patients and a Sunday spike for pediatrics. As with seasonality, an index factor should be developed to adjust the daily arrivals for the peak day of week.
3. Time of day. Depending on the adult and pediatric mix of patients, there are almost universal arrival patterns that start with declining arrival per hour until early morning, increasing to a peak rate in late morning and early afternoon, and then slowly declining through the rest of the day. It is not uncommon for pediatric patient arrivals to experience 2 peaks in late morning and early evening. An example calculation:

Annual visits = 36,500

Average daily visits 36,500/365 = 100 patients

Adjustment for seasonal peak 100 × 1.06 = 106

Adjustment for day of week 106 × 1.10 = 117

Peak period of arrival (10 AM to 7 PM) = 117 × 60% of total = 70

Peak period arrivals per hour 70/10 = 7

In this example, if the assumed average treatment room length of stay is 2 hours (120 minutes), then the peak period demand would be 840 minutes.

Establishing the treatment room capacity must be evaluated against the queuing implications resulting from random variations in the arrivals and service time. To assume that treatment space can achieve 100% average utilization guarantees intervals in which demand will exceed capacity, resulting in potentially high-risk patients waiting for care, "hall beds," and the potential of frustrated patients leaving without being seen. Establishing too low a utilization target can result in excess capacity and potentially misallocation of capital resources.

Three approaches can be used to estimate capacity. The simplest is to rely on expert judgment regarding occupancy targets. This typically ranges from 80% for low-acuity treatment spaces to 50% for trauma and higher-acuity areas. If we assumed an 80% capacity target, the required number of treatment rooms would be 18.

$$\frac{840 \text{ minutes per hour demand}}{(60 \text{ minutes } ^* 80\%) \text{capacity}} = 18 \text{ treatment spaces}$$

The most significant problem with this approach is that there is no information regarding possible waiting times and queues associated with an occupancy assumption. Conversely, there is no way to know if the target utilization percentages will result in underuse of expensive space.

Two alternative methods for addressing this project are the application of queuing theory models and stochastic simulation.[3] Queuing theory mathematical techniques were developed in the early 1900s to estimate the possible size of a queue, the wait times, and the resource utilization for systems experiencing random arrivals and service time, a common characteristic of emergency environments. There are several spreadsheet models available on the Internet to perform these calculations.

The second approach is simulation, which has the advantage of allowing to test more robust models of patient flow and arrival patterns, policy decisions regarding treatment, and the provision of detailed queuing and resource utilization patterns. Implementing this approach requires significant time and background data.

One common benchmark used in the early planning of space is the ratio of annual visits to treatment spaces. Organizations, such as the ED Benchmarking Alliance, report operational statistics for a large sample of US EDs. One of the data points is the ratio of current annual visits to treatment spaces. This ratio is computed for groups of EDs based on increments of 20,000 annual visits. The most recent ratios of visits to treatment space reports ratios ranging from 1300 to 1600 visits per treatment space.[4] It is important to remember that this is a ratio of "what is," not "what should be." Many EDs are currently experiencing overcrowding and significant peak queuing at the ratios reported in study. A review of 30 recent ED planning studies by one of the authors of this article found a ratio in the 1300 to 1400 visits as a target, with significant differences between teaching/trauma center and general community EDs (F. Zilm, unpublished data, 2019).

Once the number of treatment spaces is established, other areas, including waiting, triage, imaging, charting, supplies, and staff areas, should be developed into a comprehensive list of net square footage areas. Consideration of space to accommodate key diagnostic and support services, including imaging, laboratory, and pharmacy, should be undertaken in this phase. The most significant space, capital, and operational cost component is typically imaging. Radiographic imaging has been a standard component of emergency services. Inclusion of CT must be considered based on demand and the physical proximity to CTs located in other services. Most emergency services with 50,000 or more annual visits has CT capability within the department. Diagnostic ultrasound may also be provided within the ED. A less common element, but important for stroke and other patients, is MRI. At this point in time it is not common to include dedicated MRI capability within the ED, but shell and/or plans for addition of this service through an addition to the department should be addressed during the design.

Clinical laboratory services considerations should include the quick transport of specimens to the appropriate "stat" or other laboratory components and for the accommodation of expanding "point-of-care" testing. A staging area for pneumatic tube links to the laboratory, inclusion of satellite laboratory instruments, and "point-of-care" testing equipment and supplies. This is typically not a large area, but should including sinks, counter space, and computer access.

Inclusion of satellite pharmacies has become a more common component of a large visit volume ED. This can provide a base for a clinical pharmacologist, the delivery medications to the ED, and for the provision of "first dosage" prescriptions for patients. Patient medication dispensing machines can also be provided to supply initial patient doses.

Finally, total nontreatment space needs are added to treatment space needs (estimated by one of the methods listed previously) to yield a net usable space requirement. This sum of net usable space, is then converted into an estimate of the total dgsf needed through the application of "grossing factor" multiplier. Samples of recently completed departments have found that this ratio average 1.6.[5] If a space program listing identifies 10,000 total net square feet of usable space, the resulting estimated departmental gross area would be 16,000 dgsf. Analyses of recent EDs have shown an average of 750 dgsf per treatment space.[6]

All health care facilities must obtain approval for their architectural plans from the designated agency in their state. This agency is often referred to as the "Authority Having Jurisdiction," or AHJ. Most states use a version of space guidelines and minimum standards developed by the Health Facilities Guideline Institute.[7] These guidelines identify minimum room sizes, components that must be included in the department, and basic proximities of space elements. Some states also have a Certificate of Need program that may require applicants to meet target use goals, such as visits per treatment space. The AHJ can approve variations from the space standards if a compelling argument can be presented. Each department should evaluate special needs, such as behavioral care, isolation of infectious patients, unique surge event demands, and other requirement to determine if unique characteristics justify appealing for special space needs.

SPECIAL CONSIDERATIONS: ACADEMIC AND TERTIARY CENTERS

Some special considerations apply when designing an ED for an academic medical center, or a tertiary medical center. Academic medical center EDs provide training to a variety of medical learners, including residents, fellows, and students from medical, advanced practice, nursing, social work, pharmacy, and other schools. Additional workspace beyond what would be planned for a community site should be incorporated to accommodate these medical learners, which may include charting workstations at bedside and in staff collaboration areas. In addition, ED rooms, particularly resuscitation bays and trauma bays, may need to be sized larger than their community equivalents to accommodate medical learners. Moreover, because of the teaching function of these treatment spaces, throughput time may be slower than in an otherwise comparable community hospital, and so capacity determination should factor in this possibility. Classroom, workrooms, lockers, and break space also may be affected by the scale of educational activities. Similarly, design of EDs at tertiary medical centers should also take into account the workspace and treatment space needed for multidisciplinary care of complex or high-acuity patients.

CONSIDERING ALTERNATIVE OPERATIONAL MODELS

In addition to fundamental parameters such as projected patient volumes, staffing requirements, and institutional space and budget constraints, ED design must also take into account the operational models anticipated for the new space. Traditional ED workflows processed patients sequentially for patient flow: patients were checked in, registered, and triaged, then waited until a room and provider were available, and then taken to a room. Traditional ED design tended to reflect this processing model, with discrete spaces for check-in and registration, triage, waiting, and sometimes uniform treatment spaces for all patient types. Persistent difficulties with ED crowding[8–10] has led to renewed emphasis on strategies to increase care efficiency by using novel operational models.[11,12] These new models, along with technical innovations, such as mobile registration workstations, have introduced considerable variability between EDs in how patients are processed, particularly during early phases of care. The design of an ED should consider the flow model that is anticipated to be used, while also allowing for flexibility for future potential process model changes.

Of note, adopting any of the operational models listed in the following sections will directly impact variables that drive the calculation of treatment room capacity. For example, including a discharge lounge in the design will reduce the treatment room length of stay. Also, including a provider-in-triage will reduce the patient arrivals per hour needing a treatment room (as a subset will be discharged from the triage space). As such, the steps of determining capacity and adopting alternative operational models should be considered iterative. Each process step directly affects the other.

Split Flow

Split flow patient processing, or streaming, is an ED management model whereby patients are stratified based on their anticipated needs into different care pathways that are designed to optimize efficient care for patients of varying needs.[12,13] The most common type of split flow processing is a fast-track system, which divides patients by Emergency Severity Index (ESI) levels, with ESI 4 and 5 patients (for example) being routed to a fast track, and other ESI levels being routed into the main ED. Other types of split flow systems use the need for a bed (eg, ESI 4, 5, and "vertical ESI 3s" comprising one stream), the need for diagnostic testing, or the need for advanced imaging. Split flow has been shown to reduce wait times and lengths of stay, and particularly in the form of fast-track systems, has now been widely adopted in EDs in the United States.[14]

Design of contemporary EDs should thus consider whether a split flow system will be used, and if so, what form it will take. Key principles among split flow systems are that the space and resources of a nurse-staffed bed should not be used for patients who do not benefit from them, that patients who do not require an ED bed (as opposed to a chair or wheelchair) actually receive less-efficient care if they are placed in a bed, and that proximity to frequently used resources (eg, plain radiography) and the ED point of entry/exit are important to optimize efficiency along the patient stream requiring fewer resources.

It bears mentioning that as urgent care centers and standalone EDs have emerged in recent years, patient populations presenting to full-service EDs, particularly academic and tertiary care centers, appear to have skewed toward sicker patients with higher average resource needs.[15,16] Workflow planning and ED design should anticipate this trend, with flexibility for any low-resource split flow space to serve the needs of sicker patients should the future needs of the ED require it.

Immediate Bedding

A second major development in recent years has been the adoption of immediate bedding (also known as "direct bedding," "pull-'till-full," or "closing the waiting room"), wherein patients are taken immediately to an ED room or treatment space on check-in, and are triaged, registered, and evaluated in the treatment space.[17–20] There may be design implications from this process model, in that there is potentially less need for triage evaluation rooms. However, whether this is so depends on the match between projected patient input and the capacity of the ED being designed. Even in well-functioning EDs using immediate bedding, there may be times when patient demand outstrips available ED rooms, in which case a space for triage is necessary.

Advanced Triage and Provider-In-Triage

Advanced triage and provider-in-triage are strategies that have been adopted to smooth patient flow by maximizing the utility of the patient experience at the beginning of the visit. Advanced triage refers to the ability of triage nurses to begin workups (eg, laboratory tests, radiologic studies) or initiate focused treatment (eg, breathing treatments) based on established protocols. Provider-in-triage extends this technique by placing a physician or advanced practice provider to provide an initial evaluation simultaneous to triage, potentially allowing expedited workups or discharge from triage and shortening average length of stay.[21,22] The design implication from this process model is to have a triage space that allows for private evaluations and space to perform treatments, phlebotomy, electrocardiograms, and the like.

Results-Waiting Rooms/Discharge Lounges

A final development used to enhance patient flow is the use of ED "results-waiting" rooms or "discharge lounges." These are spaces for patients who require results before they can be safely discharged, but do not require a bed or ongoing treatment or monitoring. Use of such spaces allows new patients to be evaluated in the treatment space before results have returned. Ideally, such spaces will be separate from the waiting space for new patients (although this is not required), and will be in close proximity to providers to allow them to communicate results and discharge instructions once results are available.

COMPARING 3 TYPICAL DESIGN CONCEPTS

The ideal design solution should reflect the anticipated operational model for the service. The proposed site, proximity to other key services, and the potential reuse of existing space will impact the ability to match space to operations.

The difficulty in forecasting workloads and potential future changes in operational models can compromise subdividing spaces into discrete services, such as fast track, pediatric, or senior care. This is a "goodness-of-fit" dilemma. Designing for adaptability and change should be considered along with custom solutions for the initial operational plan. Universal examination room sizes and layouts, eliminating isolated clusters of treatment space, and positioning "soft space," such as administrative areas, to allow future growth of treatment areas are concepts that should be tested in the early schematic phases of design. Simple cardboard mockup of rooms and clusters of spaces should be used to test divergent solutions to the space program elements.

There are currently 3 typical organizational models for medium to large (more than 40,000 annual visits) emergency services: the "ballroom," "pods," and "inner core" design.

The Ballroom

This general design concept wraps as many treatment spaces as possible around a central work area. This was a common design used in the early development of EDs. A primary anticipated advantage of this approach is the visibility into the treatment spaces from charting and work areas. As treatment areas have moved from open bay configurations to larger individual patient rooms, the ability to see into more than 14 to 16 treatment areas from a single work zone becomes compromised. A second common problem in ballroom configurations is the amount of space in the central core area as the number of rooms increase. This can impact the ability of a design to fit within the targeted departmental gross square feet. Possible solutions to these problems include the development of multiple ballroom clusters and subdividing the configuration into 2 or more core workstation areas.

One significant operational advantage of this configuration is the ability to incrementally staff up and down to respond to the daily flow of patients into the service and to assign the treatment areas into groupings that match team staffing patterns. A logical expansion of this concept to meet future growth should be considered in the initial planning (**Table 1**).

Pods

One alternative to the ballroom layout is clustering treatment rooms into pods of 8 to 12 rooms. Major advantages of this approach are the ability to balance support spaces to the treatment areas, reduce staff walking distances, and the ability to maintain visibility into the treatment spaces. Pods can be designated to focus on specific services, such as pediatrics, senior care, and low-acuity patients. From an operational perspective, there are key issues that should be considered in approach. Among the most significant are the strategies for opening and closing individual pods throughout the day. Maintaining a balanced nurse-to-patient ratio is difficult during transition periods in patient census. Territoriality in a service can also potentially interfere in achieving full utilization, particularly in an academic teaching hospital environment. A third issue is avoiding duplication of supplies and equipment (**Table 2**).

Table 1
Design concept: "Ballroom" core layout

Design Concept: "Ballroom" Core Layout	Advantages	Disadvantages
	Good visibility into examination rooms Centralization of supply/utilities Ability to monitor public/emergency medical services entries	Loss of visualization into rooms in configurations of more than 16 rooms Large central "core" areas disproportionate to needs Inability to cohort-isolate infectious patients

Table 2
Design concept: "pod" configuration

Design Concept: "Pod" Configuration	Advantages	Disadvantages
	Short walking distances to examination rooms Balance of support space to patient care areas Potential subspecialization of pods to patient care needs Ability to cohort-isolate patients	Complex staffing during daily visit cycles Duplication of support services in pods Limited visualization between pods Limited control of patient/family movement

Table 3
Design concept: linear inner core configuration

Design Concept: Linear Inner Core Configuration	Advantages	Disadvantages
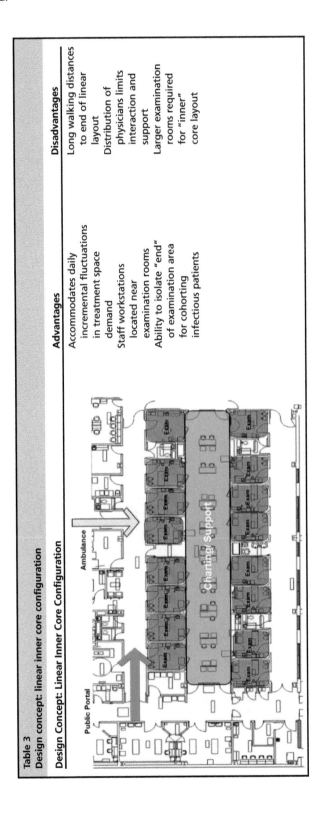	Accommodates daily incremental fluctuations in treatment space demand Staff workstations located near examination rooms Ability to isolate "end" of examination area for cohorting infectious patients	Long walking distances to end of linear layout Distribution of physicians limits interaction and support Larger examination rooms required for "inner" core layout

Inner Core

A third model that has been adopted is a linear strategy that places treatment spaces with dual room entry wrapped around an interior work corridor, with patients and family accessing the treatment rooms along an outside corridor and staff accessing treatment space through the staff work area. A variation of this concept is to abandon the interior work area and have a linear layout with corridors and work spaces similar to the ballroom concept.

This approach has the advantage of allowing incremental growth in census with less potential staffing miss-matches, as in the pod design. With proper site planning, this approach also allows for a future expansion that is consistent with the overall organization of the service. Minimizing cross-traffic of patients, family, and staff can also provide a barrier to cross contamination and the ability to cohort high-risk infectious patients. A major disadvantage of the inner core version of this concept is the need to have larger treatment rooms because of the dual entries. A second concern expressed by facilities that have implemented this approach is the isolation of the staff from other activities in the ED. Finally, this layout may also result in significant staff walking distances if workstations are intentionally consolidated for collaboration or education (**Table 3**).

INCORPORATING EVENT-SCENARIO PLANNING

An important potential emergency service demand that is frequently overlooked during the planning and design process is the impact of man-made or natural events that can create surges in volume, security risks, or other unique considerations.[23] Each department should work with their appropriate safety team to assess potential risks and determine how future plans could respond. The range of events will vary by geographic region, urban settings, and other variables. Examples of strategies that have been used include the following:

- Provision of dual headwalls in treatment spaces to accommodate potential surge volume events.
- The ability to segregate a cluster of treatment stations, with direct access from the outside, to provide "cohort" management of high-risk infectious patients.
- Oversizing the ambulance entry area to serve as a triage receiving point for surge, or security needs, events.
- The ability to quickly convert the ambulance entry, garage, or other adjacent space into a mass decontamination zone.
- Provision of concealed medical gas outlets in consultation, office, and waiting area for patient care use in a major event.
- Site access control points to restrict public vehicular access during major events presenting security or volume control needs for the emergency service.
- Blast mitigation design strategies.

SUMMARY

A doctor can bury his mistakes, but an architect can only advise his clients to plant vines.

—*Frank Lloyd Wright*

ED design affects more than just physical space. A well-executed design improves clinical efficiency, facilitates the provision of medical care, and can accommodate unforeseen changes in department needs. Delivering such a design can seem to be a daunting task, requiring leaders to envision department needs 5 to 10 years in the future, find solutions that accommodate competing needs and priorities, and work within practical financial and space constraints.

Early clinical input is important to generating a successful final design. Key operational considerations, such as split flow, immediate bedding, provider-in-triage, and discharge lounges drive physical design considerations. As design moves through the 5 major phases (strategic planning, space programming, schematic design, design development, and creation of construction documents), plans become more detailed, technical, and difficult to modify. During the early stages of the process, clinical staff has the most significant opportunity to incorporate novel ideas and influence the final design.

There is no ideal ED design solution. Rather, the solution should be tailored to the anticipated operational model for the specific department, and will be a function of the proposed site, the proximity to other key services, and the potential reuse of existing space. This article presents several design concepts (ballroom, pod, inner core), each with potential advantages and disadvantages.

ED design is neither easy nor simple. However, following a rigorous design process can mitigate the need for a department to "plant vines" to mask the clinical inefficiencies, operational work-arounds, unforeseen space needs, or rising patient volumes that will invariably arise.

DISCLOSURE

K.D. Marshall is partially supported by a grant from the Greenwall Foundation's Making a Difference program for clinical ethics research unrelated to this article's content.

REFERENCES

1. Zilm F, Crane J, Roche KT. New directions in emergency service operations and planning. J Ambul Care Manage 2010;33(4):296–306.
2. Taylor L, Nayak S. Goldratt's theory applied to the problems associated with an emergency department at a hospital. Adm Sci 2012;2(4):235–49.
3. Xavier G, Crane J, Follen M, et al. Using poisson modeling and queuing theory to optimize staffing and decrease patient wait time in the emergency department. Open J Emerg Med 2018;06(03):54–72.
4. Emergency department performance measures, initial report. Madison, WI: Emergency Department Benchmarking Alliance; 2018. Available at: https://www.edbenchmarking.org.
5. Area calculations & net: gross ratios in hospital design, preliminary report. College Station, TX: Texas A&M Center for Health Systems and Design, College of Architecture; 2012.
6. Zilm F, Augustine JJ, Strickler J. Emergency department facility design. In: Strauss RW, Mayer TA, editors. Strauss and Mayer's emergency department management. New York: McGraw-Hill Education Medical; 2014. p. 171–9.
7. The Facilities Guidelines Institute:Dallas, Texas. Guidelines for design and construction of hospitals 2018.
8. Morley C, Unwin M, Peterson GM, et al. Emergency department crowding: a systematic review of causes, consequences and solutions. PLoS One 2018;13(8):e0203316.
9. Moskop JC, Geiderman JM, Marshall KD, et al. Another look at the persistent moral problem of emergency department crowding. Ann Emerg Med 2019;74(3):357–64.

10. Chang AM, Cohen DJ, Lin A, et al. Hospital strategies for reducing emergency department crowding: a mixed-methods study. Ann Emerg Med 2018;71(4): 497–505.e4.
11. Wiler JL, Gentle C, Halfpenny JM, et al. Optimizing emergency department front-end operations. Ann Emerg Med 2010;55(2):142–60.e1.
12. Farley HL, Kwun R. Emergency department crowding: high impact solutions. Emergency Medicine Practice Committee of the American College of Emergency Medicine. 2016. Available at: https://www.acep.org/globalassets/sites/acep/media/crowding/empc_crowding-ip_092016.pdf. Accessed October 7, 2019.
13. Jensen K. The patient flow advantage: how hardwiring hospital-wide flow drives competitive performance. Gulf Breeze (NC): Fire Starter Pub; 2015.
14. Arya R, Wei G, McCoy JV, et al. Decreasing length of stay in the emergency department with a split emergency severity index 3 patient flow model. Acad Emerg Med 2013;20(11):1171–9.
15. Peterson SM, Harbertson CA, Scheulen JJ, et al. Trends and characterization of academic emergency department patient visits: a five-year review. Acad Emerg Med 2019;26(4):410–9.
16. Poon SJ, Schuur JD, Mehrotra A. Trends in visits to acute care venues for treatment of low-acuity conditions in the United States from 2008 to 2015. JAMA Intern Med 2018;178(10):1342–9.
17. Bertoty DA, Kuszajewski ML, Marsh EE. Direct-to-room: one department's approach to improving ED throughput. J Emerg Nurs 2007;33(1):26–30.
18. Tanabe P, Gisondi MA, Medendorp S, et al. Should you close your waiting room? Addressing ED overcrowding through education and staff-based participatory research. J Emerg Nurs 2008;34(4):285–9.
19. Ioannides KLH, Blome A, Schreyer KE. Impact of a direct bedding initiative on left without being seen rates. J Emerg Med 2018;55(6):850–60.
20. Basile J, Youssef E, Cambria B, et al. A novel approach to addressing an unintended consequence of direct to room: the delay of initial vital signs. West J Emerg Med 2018;19(2):254–8.
21. Partovi SN, Nelson BK, Bryan ED, et al. Faculty triage shortens emergency department length of stay. Acad Emerg Med 2001;8(10):990–5.
22. Holroyd BR, Bullard MJ, Latoszek K, et al. Impact of a triage liaison physician on emergency department overcrowding and throughput: a randomized controlled trial. Acad Emerg Med 2007;14(8):702–8.
23. Zilm F. Designing for emergencies. Integrating operations and adverse-event planning. Health Facil Manage 2010;23(11):39–42.

Lean Process Improvement in the Emergency Department

Lorna M. Breen, MD[a], Richard Trepp Jr, MD[a,b],
Nicholas Gavin, MD, MBA, MS[a],*

KEYWORDS

- Lean • Process improvement • Patient flow • Emergency department operations
- Six sigma

KEY POINTS

- Lean is a collection of methodologies aimed at eliminating waste in any process and can readily be applied to emergency department (ED) care.
- Studies have shown improvement in multiple areas of emergency care (such as door-to-provider time, patient satisfaction scores, and patient length of stay in the ED) using Lean methodologies.
- Best practices exist and increase the likelihood that changes implemented are robust and sustainable.

LEAN: GENERAL PRINCIPLES

The unsustainable growth of health care costs is leading to transformational change in day-to-day operations, incentives, and cost structures in the American health care system. In the resulting landscape, the application of Lean process engineering presents an opportunity to enhance efficiency, improve timeliness, and reduce costs.

Lean engineering has its origins with the Toyota Production System and has been defined as "an integrated sociotechnical system whose main objective is to eliminate waste by concurrently reducing or minimizing supplier, customer, and internal variability."[1] In other words, Lean may be defined as a system of management used to minimize process lead time, maximize utilization of available capacity, and eliminate steps that do not add value, or waste, in a process[2] (**Box 1**).

[a] Department of Emergency Medicine, Columbia University Vagelos College of Physicians and Surgeons, 622 West 168th Street, VC2 260, New York, NY 10032, USA; [b] NewYork-Presbyterian, New York, NY 10032, USA.
* Corresponding author. 622 W 168th Street, VC2-278, New York, NY 10032, USA.
E-mail address: ng2734@cumc.columbia.edu
Twitter: @lornambreen (L.M.B.); @NickGavinMD (N.G.)

Emerg Med Clin N Am 38 (2020) 633–646
https://doi.org/10.1016/j.emc.2020.05.001
0733-8627/20/© 2020 Elsevier Inc. All rights reserved.

emed.theclinics.com

Box 1
Lean general principles

Lean management principles include the following:
- Eliminating all forms of waste
- Fixing problems at their root
- Learning from the frontline
- Continuously improving
- Enhancing value flow
- Empowering frontline staff to "stop the line" when an error is recognized and to create the solution, as they are the subject matter experts

---

LEAN APPLICATIONS IN HEALTH CARE

Rotter and colleagues[3] described 2 key components to Lean management in health care: Lean philosophy (the underlying Lean principles discussed earlier, including the idea of continuous improvement) and Lean activities (assessment and improvement focused). Lean assessment activities, which we will detail later include Gemba walk, value stream mapping, creation and integration of A3s, and rapid process improvement workshops or rapid improvement events (**Box 2**). Lean improvement activities include creation of standard work, 5S organizing, "stop the line" techniques or Andon, and daily visual management.

Gemba Walk

Gemba, the Japanese term for "the real place," is the place where value is created.[4] In health care, this can be in the clinic, the laboratory, the radiology suite, or in the back office. A Gemba walk refers to going to that place of work and observing. This activity can inform both decision-making and experiment design. Going to the Gemba may be most important when decision-makers hold preconceived notions about the way forward.

Examples of Gemba walks described in the literature include use as a general management strategy, as a tool for assessing and improving laboratory turn-around-time,[5] improving safe medication administration,[6] and enhancing efficiency in an outpatient clinic.[7]

The power of the Gemba walk is in the ability of project stakeholders to follow the patient's journey or observe the staff's actual workflow and then engage in honest dialogue about options for going forward.

Box 2
Lean applications in health care

Lean assessment activities include the following:
- Gemba walk
- Value stream mapping
- Creation and integration of A3s
- Rapid process improvement workshops or rapid improvement events

Lean improvement activities include
- Creation of standard work
- "Stop the line" techniques or Andon
- 5S
- Daily visual management

Value Stream Mapping

Another key principle of Lean methodologies is enhancing the flow of value and eliminating non–value-added steps. A value stream mapping exercise first defines the concrete steps in a process and then evaluates each step, and delay between steps, in terms of whether or not it adds value to the consumer. In many health care examples, the consumer is the patient, but at times it is also providers or staff. Typically, a value stream mapping exercise starts with a map of current state. Non–value-added steps and delays between steps are then identified and that information is used to inform creation of an ideal or future state process that eliminates non–value-added steps and reduces delays between steps.

Value stream mapping can be used to redesign any patient flow process, such as intake into or flow through an emergency department (ED). But it is important to recognize that the same methodology can be applied to the flow of information, equipment, or medications. **Fig. 1** is an example of value stream mapping in the rapid medical evaluation area of the ED.

A3

One strategy for new initiatives is the creation of an A3. A3 refers to a size of paper (11″ by 17″) that is (in the context of Lean) formatted in a way that helps frame a problem in a structured manner and address root causes. A3s' content varies, but they typically include a project's title and owner, the background of the problem, a description of current conditions, a definition of the goal or target conditions, an analysis describing root causes of the issue, a list of countermeasures, an implementation plan, and description of follow-up. The A3 thus helps to visualize the plan-do-study/check-act cycle.

A3s have many applications in health care; for example, they can be used at the project level or for tracking of a committee's broader work. **Fig. 2** is an example of an A3.

Rapid Process Improvement Workshops or Rapid Improvement Events

Structured events, often called rapid improvement events, or Kaizen events, can be organized in order to bring stakeholders together to design and rapidly experiment with changes to a given process. Within the event, various Lean assessment methodologies are used to inform the event's progress. Often the goal of such events is to eliminate workarounds or ambiguity and create standard work. Interdisciplinary, team-based problem solving is key to the success of rapid improvement events.

Andon or Stop the Line

Setting the standard that anyone can "stop the line" (ie, halt routine work until a quality issue is addressed) is another important aspect of Lean. In health care, it is also a strategy that has been deployed in operating rooms, clinics, EDs, and intensive care units. Often in high-pressure, fast-paced environments, errors can occur if a process is relying on one person's ability to identify a potential problem. Because health care is a team sport, giving anyone who recognizes a problem the ability to "stop the line" or "pull the Andon cord" is both meaningful and impactful.

5S

A standardized method for organizing workspace, 5S is shorthand for Sort, Set in order, Shine, Standardize, and Sustain. The most frequent application of the 5S tool in health care is in supplies and equipment storage. Sorting reduces the time to find an item. Setting in order makes it possible for an individual's work to be functionally easy

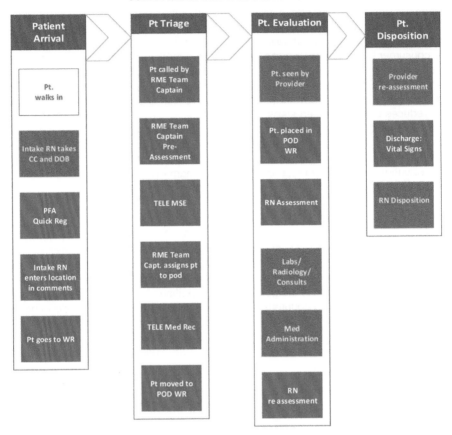

RME Redesign: Patient Process
Value Added and Non Value Added

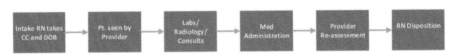

Fig. 1. Rapid medical evaluation redesign: Patient process value added and non value added.

from a movement standpoint. Shining, or cleaning the workspace, makes it more safe and efficient to navigate. Standardization applies to the first 3 steps for all work areas at a facility or within an organization. Finally, sustainment involves implementing 5S across an enterprise. **Fig. 3** is an example of the results of the 5S tool.

LEAN IN EMERGENCY DEPARTMENTS

Lean methodologies have been deployed in EDs in many domains. Although often inspired by adverse patient safety events or directives from the executive suite, the

Date/Version: August 30, 2017   Owner:
                                                       Sponsor(s):
Title: Team:

Background:	Recommendation/Proposed Changes:
Current State:	
	Action Items:
	What Who When
Problem Statement:	
Goal/Aim:	
Analysis of Problem:	Measures and Follow-up:

Fig. 2. Example of an A3.

Lean Activities: 5S

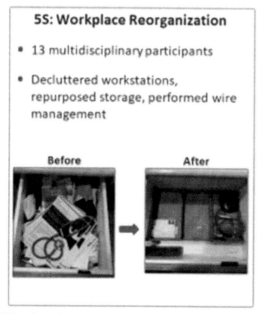

Fig. 3. Example of S5 tool results.

most successful improvement initiatives frequently are derived from a team's desire to compete with themselves and pushed to new heights with current resources. In EDs, project owners may be nursing or physician leaders, but it is important to recognize when ancillary service stakeholders should take ownership and drive change within their domains. Regardless of the initiative, an early first step is identifying all stakeholders involved in the process, and a key next step is recognizing their incentives to change.

Soliciting ideas for improvement is a critical skill for an ED leader. One unique approach that has been used to gather suggestions is the creation "Kaizen portal" where ED residents and attendings can submit suggestions that are evaluated and (when able) implemented by the ED leadership group.[8] Another group required EM residents to submit "Health Systems" logs with observations of the Health Care System or patient safety reports.[9] Regardless of methodology, engagement with frontline staff through all phases of improvement is key to a project's success (**Box 3**).

CHANGES RESULTING FROM LEAN EVENTS
Improving the Intake Process

Streamlining the steps from when a patient arrives to when the patient is seen by a provider is an important consideration in ED Lean redesign. Registration and the triage process are common areas of focus in the intake process.[10] Bedside registration is often used to minimize the number of stops a patient has to make after entering the ED.[11–14] Some of the changes that have been made to triage are reassigning movement of arriving patients to someone other than the triage nurse to avoid taking them away from triage,[15] moving the location of the charts and equipment to the most convenient location for the triage nurse,[16] eliminating non–value-added activities from triage,[17] assigning an additional nurse to triage during peak hours, using nursing order protocols in triage when appropriate,[18] and streamlining the nursing triage questionnaire.[19] Bedside triage, also called "direct bedding," is an approach frequently used to eliminate unnecessary steps in patient flow. This best practice embraces triage as a process, not a place.[10–12,14,18] One group enabled this process by breaking triage into 3 phases, "15-second triage" done before the patient is place in a room, "quick triage" documenting critical information such as vital signs and allergies, and "data triage" including information such as smoking history.[20] Other groups have found combined nurse and provider triage to be useful.[19] One ED improved door-to-provider times by giving providers the option to triage with nursing staff, with the potential goal of being able to discharge some patients directly from the triage location, having triage nurse-driven orders only be applied to patients who were not

---

Box 3
Major themes in improved care as a result of applying Lean principles in emergency departments

Major themes in improved care as a result of applying Lean principles in EDs are as follows:
   Improving the intake process
   Maximizing efficiency of care from time of provider evaluation to time of disposition
   Minimizing steps
   Segmenting the patient population into specialized care areas
   Standardizing work for each member of ED team
   Streamlining diagnostic testing
   Standardizing the admission process

expected to see a physician within an hour, having the emergency provider assess patients arriving by ambulance in a hallway instead of waiting for a bed to be free, and informing individual providers their door-to-provider times.[21]

Maximizing Efficiency from Time of Provider Evaluation to Time of Disposition

There have been a wide variety of changes described to try to make ED care more efficient. Changing patient distribution to a round-robin assignment system, adjusting staff breaks to permit better coverage of the ED, and moving frequently used medications to the top drawers in the medicine cart were changes made by one ED based on staff input.[22] A unique approach to improving patient flow through the department involved having individuals in a remote location monitor ED patients around the clock electronically. Those individuals monitored processes such as the wait time to see a provider and notified the physician or nurse when they saw delays.[23] Creation of a surge protocol that was based on reports every 2 hours of certain indicators (such as number of beds available, number of admitted patients) helped streamline flow during high-volume times at another ED.[21]

Other solutions proposed by front-line staff and used during process change events were ordering and sending laboratory and radiology tests earlier in the process, improving signage for patients entering and leaving the ED, and identifying opportunities to involve other services earlier.[13] One effective method involved having the nurse, resident, and attending get the patients' history at the same time whenever possible to reduce duplication of work and save staff time.[13] Matching nurse practitioner shifts to patient arrival times was a change made in one department.[19]

Other examples of changes made include the utilization of care coordinators to expedite appropriate admission and facilitate discharges, regular meetings between ED nursing leadership and inpatient nurse managers, switching from portable telephones to walkie-talkies to facilitate staff and physician communication and reduce noise, and rearranging use of storage spaces to make room for more computer stations.[20] One group had ED nurses use an "upstream patient flow tool" to notify the intensive care unit what patient load it could expect from the ED within a 2- to 4-hour window.[24] Communication was improved significantly by standardizing huddle schedules, including all ED staff in huddles and using the electronic tracking system and comment field to guide huddle discussions and communicate patient care plans.[18]

Minimizing Steps

Many of the changes put into place during Lean events involved minimizing unnecessary steps for members of the ED staff. One ED reduced nurses' average miles walked per shift from 8 to 11 miles to 3 to 6 miles by creating a central supply room and by creating standardized bedside carts and procedure carts, which eliminated the need to have specialty rooms.[25] One department highlighted the excess walking being done by the ED secretaries by using pedometers. Realizing that they were walking an average of 6 miles per shift showed the need to change their workflow so that they could be readily available to answer the phone.[20] By dividing the ED into sections that correlated with nursing assignments, steps between patients were minimized.[20] Another ED improved metrics during a Lean event that involved standardizing intravenous carts, reorganizing stock carts so that 90% of the most used stock were within steps of the patient with all physician-required material to the patient's right.[26] Yet another standard procedure cart is placed in each procedure room so that providers would not need to leave the room each time to gather supplies.[27]

Segmenting the Patient Population into Specialized Care Areas

Creating different care locations for different types of patients (often called "split flow") is a common theme in many EDs that use Lean methodologies, particularly as ED volumes grow. Examples of care area changes include ED that created a rapid triage and treatment system in which a physician was immediately adjacent to triage nurses to address triage questions and treat Emergency Severity Index 4 and 5 patients; a fast track area for patients with low-acuity complaints[10,21]; a separate rapid assessment and disposition area for patient who do not require beds[28–30]; a separate physical area of the ED (which was previously inefficiently used) for a rapid medical evaluation unit[31,32]; a "flex-pod" that could be used for various types of patient care designed from underutilized ED space[33]; separate zones for complex, medium, and fast patients[34,35]; and a "Care Initiation area" (carved out of ED space not being used any more) of 16 chairs and 4 bays for patients to come directly to that area rather than wait in the waiting room.[36] A "flow nurse" position that was converted from another nursing position made sure patients were placed in the appropriate care area.[16]

Standardizing Work for Each Member of the Emergency Department Team

Giving charge nurses the responsibility to monitor and facilitate the flow of patients to providers was also found to be helpful.[10] One ED rewrote job descriptions for everyone in the department, being explicit about what the exact roles and responsibilities were for each person.[20] Another clearly defined the roles of specific nurses (such as charge nurse, primary nurse, fast track nurse) as well as nursing assistant, flow physician, and communication physician.[18] Redefining responsibilities of nurses, nurses assistants, and the intake coordinator streamlined care in one case.[13] One group established a "communication specialist" role to coordinate incoming referrals and communication regarding ED patients (current or expected) with other providers (such as primary care providers and in-hospital providers). They also created an automated phone system that allowed callers to be routed directly to the communication specialist.[34]

Streamlining Testing

Improving the use of point-of-care laboratory tests has been found to increase efficiency of care.[10] Encouraging the team to stop sending extra tubes of blood to the laboratories "just in case" helped improve laboratory efficiency, which in turn helped drive down ED length of stay.[16] Having stable, ambulatory patients go to outpatient radiology and phlebotomy with a "priority pass" to ensure timely testing freed up ED nurses to focus on sicker patients.[18] Changing computed tomography (CT) protocols such that oral contrast was not automatically given to patients receiving abdominal CTs led to a reduction in time to receive a CT scan.[16,37] Other successful changes to the CT scan process included having CT techs pull patients, shifting CT tech hours to better cover busiest hours of the day, using wireless communication devices to improve communication between radiology and ED staff, and giving CT techs daily scorecards of their own individual performance with CT turnaround times.[37]

Standardizing the Admissions Process

Standardizing work and streamlining operations to admit a patient from the ED were the goals of several successful quality improvement initiatives.[38,39] Measuring time stamps around each step (eg, paging the admitting team, creation and placement of an order set including the minimum orders necessary for the nursing supervisor to assign an appropriate bed, and development of a handoff tool faxed from ED nurse to floor nurse) allowed standardization of the admissions process.[39] In order to expedite patient admissions, one group created a set of orders that could be used for patients who were stable and ready to go to the floor.[20] Another eliminated multiple steps in the process between when the ED physician decided to admit a patient and when the patient left the ED.[15] Other efforts to standardize the admission process include the creation of inclusion and exclusion criteria for admitting services, improving the electronic bed request form to include required information more consistently, defining standard work for each person involved in the admitting process, standardizing criteria for steps in care that needed to occur before admission versus those that could wait for after admission, creation of a standardized sign-out tool to be used by the ED provider giving report to the inpatient provider, use of a scorecard indicating potential deterioration of admitted patients (which helped inpatient teams determine which patients to see in the ED before admission),[40] and the creation of physician and nursing handover checklists in the Electronic Medical Record.[41]

USING METRICS TO MONITOR SUCCESS

There is a wide range of metrics that EDs have measured and improved on using Lean processes (**Box 4**).

SUSTAINABILITY AND POTENTIAL PITFALLS

Although Lean events help departments decide which changes to make, it does not help address the need to change culture in order to sustain those changes. There are some recurring recommendations made about making sure that changes that are made are sustained.

Getting Frontline Staff Buy-In

Making sure to get staff input and buy-in is key to success in any process change. One way to do that is to have staff take ownership by participating in the evaluation of current state, design of interventions, and ultimate decisions. A strong leader is necessary but not sufficient for end-user buy-in.[20] Focusing on team work and suggesting that staff think of patients as neighbors, friends, and family may help appeal to human factors in the workplace and can improve buy-in to change.[11] Other suggestions to improve staff buy-in include the following: making sure communication and in-servicing about new process takes place, initiating the new processes during off-peak times and in the presence of process owners and executive staff, including members from all shifts in the process, and developing clinical "champions" and midlevel managers. One group asked the staff members to present the work that they had done to the hospital board. Each slide was presented by the staff member who had championed that change in the process.[36]

Ensuring that Leadership Is Engaged

Engagement of leadership from other departments outside of the ED's control (such Radiology and Admitting) can be vital to implementing changes. Having engaged leadership who are patient and present on the unit and who set and focus on clear goals that do not change as the process changes occur improves the chance of success.[10] Support from hospital and ED leadership is critical to success with process change. Participation of hospital leaders help with interdepartmental collaboration, ensure alignment with broader organizational goals, and are necessary to remove barriers to adoption of Lean interventions. One study that compared various EDs' Lean

Box 4
Metrics to monitor success

Ambulance Diversion[29,30,36]

Patient walkouts:
   Patient leaving before being seen[10,19–21,23,26,28,30,35,36,40,44–48]
   Patient leaving before completing treatment[29]

Triage:
   Door-to-triage times[48,49]
   Number of ESI 3 patients waiting for triage[51]
   Number of low-acuity patients awaiting triage[17]
   Nurse-to-patient ratio at triage[50]

Patient movement through the department:
   Triage-to-provider time[12,14]
   Door-to-room time[35]
   Time to see a provider[10–12,20,25,26,28,31,35,47–49]
   Registration-to-disposition times[49]
   Doctor-to-disposition times[32]
   Time from decision to admit to transfer to floor[14]
   Time between "bed ready" and patient arrival on the inpatient unit[54]

Improved testing:
   Arrival to first-order, radiograph, laboratory collected[33]
   Variation in common laboratory turnaround times[43]
   Rates of laboratory specimen hemolysis[42]
   Laboratory turnaround times[43,55]
   Transportation of ED patients for plain films[56]
   Time from CT ordered to CT complete[57]

Length of stay (LOS):
   Overall LOS[12,13,16,20,21,23,25,28–30,32,35,36,45,52]
   LOS for low-acuity[16,27,31,46] and mid-acuity[53] patients
   LOS for discharged patients[34]
   LOS for admitted patients[34,39,40]

ED crowding:
   Use of hallway beds[33]
   ED boarding time[38]
   Overall ED crowding[40]

Provider productivity:
   Patients per MD hour[49]

Patient satisfaction:
   Overall patient satisfaction scores[11,13,20,26,34,36,38,44,45,47]

Increased ED patient volume[11,13,20,36,45]

Impact to staff:
   Cooperation among ED staff members[11]
   Increased staff satisfaction scores and decreased turnover[22]

ED noise levels[20]

Improved safety:
   Streamlined medicine reconciliation process[58]
   Communication errors between ED and inpatient teams[41]

Abbreviation: ESI, Emergency Severity Index.

Data from Refs.[10–14,16,17,19–23,25–36,38–58]

Box 5

Suggested practices for making and sustaining changes

Suggested practices for making and sustaining changes include the following:
  Get staff buy-in
  Make sure other departments are included
  Ensure that leadership is engaged
  Address naysayers
  Give timely feedback
  Make changes as needed

---

projects showed that the greatest successes were seen when both frontline staff and management were heavily involved in the process and when Lean principles were strictly adhered to.[52]

Addressing Naysayers

It is also important to have a strategy to address naysayers, as even the best strategies can draw detractors. One principle is to ensure that those who disagree with process improvements have an opportunity to discuss their concerns openly before implementation. However, once a process change with demonstrable benefits has been started, it is important to ensure compliance. One potential avenue to ensuring this is to obtain commitments from a hospital CEO and ED medical director that noncompliance would not be accepted before implementing a change.[11]

Giving Timely Feedback

Leaders need to review and share data regularly (some recommend daily!) as well as round in the ED every day during the pilot and during the change. One group implemented a daily management system that involved a brief huddle with frontline staff to check on the standard work that had been implemented and review timestamps and LOS metrics to reinforce and track use of the standard work.[39] Using a communication board in the department with current metrics, areas in which improvement has occurred, list of target goals, action item list, and comment box (including complaints about the processes) reviewed by the management team daily is one way that has been found to keep staff engaged in process change.[29] When ED clinicians and staff are eager to see performance metrics that are posted monthly, they are more likely to be engaged in new processes.[10] Having a plan that specifies ownership for processes and changes brought about during initiatives is important to ensure that the changes are sustained.[59]

Making Changes as Needed

In cases where the new process was not followed, the leaders identified and logged barriers so that leadership could further investigate the most common causes (**Box 5**).

SUMMARY

Lean methodologies are a collection of tools that can be used to maximize the efficiency of care in the ED. The most successful Lean projects involve buy-in from staff and leadership. There are several well-described steps that can be used to decide which issues to prioritize and how to best improve those processes. Providing ongoing and timely feedback are critical, both during and after a Lean event, and vital to increasing the success and sustainability of the project.

DISCLOSURE

The authors have no financial conflicts to disclose.

REFERENCES

1. Shah RaW P. Defining and developing measures of lean production. J Oper Manag 2007;25(4):785–805.
2. George ML, Rowlands D, Price M, et al. The lean six sigma pocket toolbook: a quick reference guideto nearly 100 tools for improving quality, speed, and complexity. McGraw-Hill; 2004.
3. Rotter T, Plishka C, Lawal A, et al. What Is lean management in health care? development of an operational definition for a cochrane systematic review. Eval Health Prof 2019;42(3):366–90.
4. Liker JK. The Toyota Way. McGraw-Hill: New York,2004.
5. Gupta S, Kapil S, Sharma M. Improvement of laboratory turnaround time using lean methodology. Int J Health Care Qual Assur 2018;31(4):295–308.
6. Manojlovich M, Chase VJ, Mack M, et al. Using A3 thinking to improve the STAT medication process. J Hosp Med 2014;9(8):540–4.
7. Lot LT, Sarantopoulos A, Min LL, et al. Using Lean tools to reduce patient waiting time. Leadersh Health Serv 2018;31(3):343–51.
8. Jacobson GH, McCoin NS, Lescallette R, et al. Kaizen: a method of process improvement in the emergency department. Acad Emerg Med 2009;16(12):1341–9.
9. Kane B, Yenser D, Barr G, et al. Capturing resident observed concerns regarding both the patient safety and the health care system: An innovative use of resident logs. West J Emerg Med 2017;18:S42.
10. Lean-driven solutions slash ED wait times, LOS. ED Manag 2012;24(12):139–41.
11. Lean-driven improvements slash wait times, drive up patient satisfaction scores. ED Manag 2012;24(7):79–81.
12. Agoritsas K, Peacock P, Legome E, et al. Applying lean to improve throughput metrics in a pediatric emergency department. Acad Emerg Med 2016;23:S62.
13. Dickson EW, Singh S, Cheung DS, et al. Application of lean manufacturing techniques in the Emergency Department. J Emerg Med 2009;37(2):177–82.
14. Kulkarni RG. Going lean in the emergency department: a strategy for addressing emergency department overcrowding. MedGenMed 2007;9(4):58.
15. Kolker A. A reader and author respond to "Going lean in the emergency department: a strategy for addressing emergency department overcrowding". Medscape J Med 2008;10(2):25 [author reply: 25].
16. Arbune A, Wackerbarth S, Allison P, et al. Improvement through Small Cycles of Change: Lessons from an Academic Medical Center Emergency Department. J Healthc Qual 2017;39(5):259–69.
17. Farley H, Hines D, Ross E, et al. A lean-based triage redesign process improves door-to-room times and decreases number of patients at triage. Ann Emerg Med 2009;54(3):S96.
18. Vashi AA, Sheikhi FH, Nashton LA, et al. Applying Lean Principles to Reduce Wait Times in a VA Emergency Department. Mil Med 2019;184(1–2):e169–78.
19. Preston-Suni K, Fleischman R, Ramon J, et al. Triage improvements reduce wait times and eliminate disparities for patients with limited english proficiency. Acad Emerg Med 2019;26:S84.
20. Lean-driven improvements eliminate waste, boost patient satisfaction in a matter of weeks. ED Manag 2013;25(12):136–9.

21. Patey C, Norman P, Araee M, et al. SurgeCon: priming a community emergency department for patient flow management. West J Emerg Med 2019;20(4):654–65.
22. Phillips J, Hebish LJ, Mann S, et al. Engaging Frontline Leaders and Staff in Real-Time Improvement. Jt Comm J Qual Patient Saf 2016;42(4):170–83.
23. Culture of safety' sets tone for improvement. ED Manag 2007;19(6):64–5.
24. Florida hospital saves 5.3 M dollars by adopting principles of lean manufacturing. Perform Improv Advis 2005;9(1):10–1, 11.
25. ED improves on already impressive wait times. ED Manag 2010;22(1):6–7.
26. Ng D, Vail G, Thomas S, et al. Applying the Lean principles of the Toyota Production System to reduce wait times in the emergency department. CJEM 2010;12(1):50–7.
27. White BA, Chang Y, Grabowski BG, et al. Using lean-based systems engineering to increase capacity in the emergency department. West J Emerg Med 2014;15(7):770–6.
28. Gardner RM, Friedman N, Bradham T, et al. Impact of revised triage approach to improving emergency department throughput for treat and release patients. Acad Emerg Med 2017;24:S157.
29. ED becomes 'lean' and cuts LBTC, LOS times. ED Manag 2008;20(4):44–5.
30. Eller A. Rapid assessment and disposition: applying LEAN in the emergency department. J Healthc Qual 2009;31(3):17–22.
31. Chartier LB, Kuipers M, Josephson T. Plenary oral presentations. CJEM 2015;17(Suppl 2):S4–88.
32. Luu AS, Cheffers M, Kearl YL, et al. LEAN in to get patients out: North project. Ann Emerg Med 2016;68(4):S21.
33. Arnold T, Buenger LE, Jensen G, et al. Lean methodology to improve patient flow through flexible space utilization. Acad Emerg Med 2018;25:S64.
34. Woodward GA, Godt MG, Fisher K, et al. Children's hospital and regional medical center emergency department patient flow–rapid process improvement (RPI). In: Chalice R, editor. Improving healthcare quality using Toyota lean production methods: 46 steps for improvement. 2nd ed. Milwaukee: Quality; 2007. p. 145–50.
35. Murrell KL, Offerman SR, Kauffman MB. Applying lean: implementation of a rapid triage and treatment system. West J Emerg Med 2011;12(2):184–91.
36. Care initiation area yields dramatic results. ED Manag 2009;21(3):28–9.
37. Humphries R, Russell PM, Pennington RJ, et al. Utilizing lean management techniques to improve emergency department radiology ct turnaround times. Ann Emerg Med 2011;58(4):S248.
38. Sroufe NS. Reducing emergency department boarding time: A quality improvement initiative. Acad Emerg Med 2014;21(5):S290.
39. Allaudeen N, Vashi A, Breckenridge JS, et al. Using lean management to reduce emergency department length of stay for medicine admissions. Qual Manag Health Care 2017;26(2):91–6.
40. Migita R, Del Beccaro M, Cotter D, et al. Emergency department overcrowding: Developing emergency department capacity through process improvement. Clin Pediatr Emerg Med 2011;12(2):141–50.
41. Mahajan P. Quality in pediatric emergency medicine: A learning curve and a curveball. Clin Pediatr Emerg Med 2011;12(2):80–90.
42. Damato C, Rickard D. Using Lean-Six Sigma to reduce hemolysis in the emergency care center in a collaborative quality improvement project with the hospital laboratory. Jt Comm J Qual Patient Saf 2015;41(3):99–107.

43. Sanders JH, Karr T. Improving ED specimen TAT using Lean Six Sigma. Int J Health Care Qual Assur 2015;28(5):428–40.

44. ED redesign improves patient flow, satisfaction. Hosp Case Manag 2013; 21(4):53–4.

45. Carstairs KL, Hollenbach KA, Shah S, et al. Improved emergency department quality metrics, patient satisfaction scores, and revenue following implementation of lean flow principles and queuing theory-based operational changes. Acad Emerg Med 2016;23:S59–60.

46. Kanzaria H, Mercer M, To J, et al. Using lean methodology to create a care pathway for low acuity emergency department patients in a safety net hospital. Acad Emerg Med 2017;24:S202–3.

47. Lisankie M, Saint-Hilaire R, Wein DA, et al. Split-improves operational flow and decreases flow emergency department layout process variation. Ann Emerg Med 2016;68(4):S89.

48. Vashi AA, Haji-Sheikhi F, Nashton LA, et al. Applying lean principles to reduce wait times in the emergency department. J Gen Intern Med 2016;31(2):S120.

49. Naik T, Duroseau Y, Zehtabchi S, et al. A structured approach to transforming a large public hospital emergency department via lean methodologies. J Healthc Qual 2012;34(2):86–97.

50. Ross E, Hines DM, Farley H, et al. A lean-based process redesign to expedite throughput of emergency severity index (ESI)-3 patients reduces the percentage of time recommended nurse to patient ratios are exceeded at triage. Acad Emerg Med 2010;17:S97.

51. Hines DM, Ross E, Farley H, et al. A lean-based process redesign intended to expedite patient throughput improves door to room times and decreases patients at triage. Acad Emerg Med 2010;17:S91.

52. Dickson EW, Anguelov Z, Vetterick D, et al. Use of lean in the emergency department: a case series of 4 hospitals. Ann Emerg Med 2009;54(4):504–10.

53. Cheffers M, Luu A, Laird D, et al. Utilization of lean healthcare principles to improve emergency department patient flow in an intermediate acuity area of a safety-net hospital. Acad Emerg Med 2016;23:S248.

54. White BA, Bravard MA, Kobayashi KJ, et al. Improving handoff efficiency for admitted patients: A multidisciplinary, lean-based approach. Am J Emerg Med 2019;37(6):1202–3.

55. White BA, Baron JM, Dighe AS, et al. Applying Lean methodologies reduces ED laboratory turnaround times. Am J Emerg Med 2015;33(11):1572–6.

56. White BA, Yun BJ, Lev MH, et al. Applying systems engineering reduces radiology transport cycle times in the emergency department. West J Emerg Med 2017;18(3):410–8.

57. Klein D, Khan V. Utilizing six sigma lean strategies to expedite emergency department CT scan throughput in a tertiary care facility. J Am Coll Radiol 2017;14(1):78–81.

58. Hummel J, Evans PC, Lee H. Medication reconciliation in the emergency department: opportunities for workflow redesign. Qual Saf Health Care 2010;19(6):531–5.

59. Rotteau L, Webster F, Salkeld E, et al. Ontario's emergency department process improvement program: the experience of implementation. Acad Emerg Med 2015;22(6):720–9.

Alternative Dispositions for Emergency Department Patients

Alice Kidder Bukhman, MD, MPH[a,b,*],
Christopher W. Baugh, MD, MBA[c], Brian J. Yun, MD, MBA, MPH[d]

KEYWORDS

- Alternative dispositions • Observation unit • Home hospital • Rapid follow-up clinic
- Evidence-based clinical pathways • Accelerated diagnostic pathways

KEY POINTS

- Use of alternative dispositions from the emergency department may help reduce emergency department crowding through increasing inpatient bed capacity.
- There is an array of alternative dispositions that can deliver equivalent outcomes at lower costs and with shorter lengths of stay and greater patient satisfaction compared with inpatient admission for select clinical conditions.
- Adoption of alternative dispositions requires institutions to build processes and resources to promote their use. These processes and resources include investments in rapid follow-up clinics, observation units, and home hospital programs, as well as development and implementation of validated evidence-based clinical pathways.

ALTERNATIVE DISPOSITIONS AS A TOOL TO TACKLE EMERGENCY DEPARTMENT CROWDING

Emergency department (ED) crowding is a continuing challenge, resulting in increased morbidity and mortality and decreased patient satisfaction. Patients with greater than 12 hours of ED boarding have been shown to have significantly higher mortality than those with shorter lengths of stay.[1] Studies have also found ED crowding is associated with delayed antibiotics and fluids in sepsis[2] and increased mortality in patients with out-of-hospital cardiac arrest.[3]

Admitted patients waiting for inpatient beds are a primary driver of ED crowding. Evidence suggests that there is a subset of these patients for whom an alternative

[a] Brigham and Women's Faulkner Emergency Department, 1153 Centre Street, Boston, MA 02130, USA; [b] Department of Emergency Medicine, Brigham and Women's Hospital, 75 Francis Street, Neville House 2nd Floor, Boston, MA 02115, USA; [c] Department of Emergency Medicine, Brigham and Women's Hospital, 75 Francis Street, Neville House 2nd Floor, Boston, MA 02115, USA; [d] Department of Emergency Medicine, Massachusetts General Hospital, 55 Fruit Street, Boston, MA 02114, USA
* Corresponding author. 1153 Centre Street, Boston, MA 02130.
E-mail address: abukhman@bwh.harvard.edu

Emerg Med Clin N Am 38 (2020) 647–661
https://doi.org/10.1016/j.emc.2020.04.004
0733-8627/20/© 2020 Elsevier Inc. All rights reserved.
emed.theclinics.com

disposition can safely and effectively replace inpatient admission, and that this may help to alleviate both hospital and ED crowding.[4]

Strategies to decrease admissions from the ED when another disposition might be reasonable include:

- Rapidly referring ED patients to outpatient diagnostics and therapies
- Hospitalizing patients in observation units using evidence-based protocolized care pathways
- Hospitalizing patients at home through home hospital programs
- Community-based interventions, such as telemedicine, emergency medical services (EMS)–directed pathways, and expanded clinic access, to avoid or bypass the ED
- Use of care coordination and policies such as the Medicare skilled nursing facility (SNF) waiver to place appropriate patients in rehabilitation facilities, bypassing inpatient admission

Adoption of these admission alternatives can be supported with evidence-based clinical pathways that support the alternative plan as safe (eg, within the acceptable standard of care), as well as patient engagement via shared decision making[5] (SDM; **Fig. 1**).

TOOLS TO SUPPORT ALTERNATIVE DISPOSITIONS: EVIDENCE-BASED CLINICAL PATHWAYS AND SHARED DECISION MAKING
Evidence-Based Clinical Pathways

Clinicians are most familiar with inpatient hospitalization as the setting for the work-up of a potentially dangerous patient complaint that remains unresolved after a standard

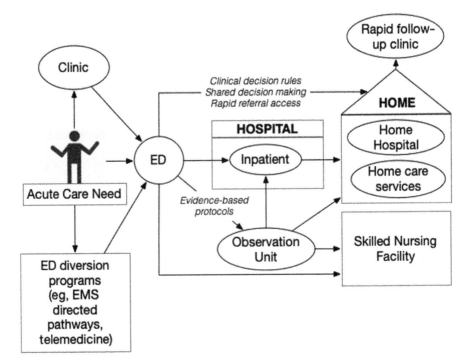

Fig. 1. Alternative dispositions.

ED visit. Clinicians and patients have little incentive to choose an alternative strategy such as observation or discharge to a rapid follow-up clinic without evidence of safety and efficacy. Creation and validation of accelerated diagnostic pathways (ADPs) and decision rules (collectively referred to as evidence-based clinical pathways) can provide this guidance and reassurance.[5] There are dozens of such validated pathways that seek to reduce unnecessary laboratory or radiology testing or admission.[5] These pathways are particularly attractive for gray-zone conditions, in which there exists clinical equipoise between different dispositions, and for which researchers have noted the greatest variation in admission decisions.[6] These protocols can help support a patient's or clinician's choice of a disposition other than inpatient admission.

There are many barriers to the acceptance of a new ADP, including a perceived loss of clinical decision-making autonomy on the part of the clinicians; lack of acceptance of the pathway among referring outpatient clinicians and specialists; questions as to the reliability of the outpatient follow-up system; and lack of agreement about whether the researcher's definition of equivalence and safety matches that of the patient, clinician, and medicolegal community.[5,7] Although there are a host of examples of validated clinical decision rules, most cannot alone promise the level of rule-out certainty that clinicians and patients may want.

Emergency physicians in the United States are typically held to a low level of risk tolerance, generally less than 1% risk of missing a serious diagnosis,[8] and few advanced diagnostic pathways can ensure that level of sensitivity. For example, a recent meta-analysis found that the widely accepted HEART (history, electrocardiography, age, risk factors, troponin) score diagnostic pathway missed 3.3% of patients with a major adverse cardiac event, raising the question of whether this level of risk is tolerable to the medical community.[9] Some conditions, such as heart failure, carry a high baseline risk of poor outcomes. An emergency physician may be reluctant to be last clinician to treat such high-risk patients before discharge, even when alternatives to inpatient admission are appropriate.[10]

Validated clinical decision rules likely offer some protection to clinicians against malpractice. One study found that, of 60 malpractice cases brought against clinicians for failure to order head computed tomography (CT) between 1972 and 2014, the 10 that were found in favor of the plaintiff all were cases in which a relevant decision rule suggested imaging or further observation.[11] Moreover, when used in conjunction with an observation unit or rapid follow-up clinic, these pathways can offer reassurance while still avoiding unnecessary hospitalizations.[5] Chest pain has probably generated the greatest number of such validated decision rules, but, here as well, most studies have shown safety when the tool is paired with an alternative disposition, such as observation or rapid clinic follow-up.[12–16] One recent study integrated use of the HEART score advanced diagnostic pathway with rapid referral to a specialty chest pain clinic, with an estimated 20% reduction in inpatient hospital health care costs.[17]

However, clinical pathways do not affect admission rates if clinicians do not know them or use them. Given the increased use of electronic health medical records, some clinicians have studied the integration of electronic clinical decision support systems (CDSSs) to standardize and promote use of validated decision rules.[18] One recent study of CDSSs with patients with pulmonary embolism found its use safely reduced inpatient admissions.[19] ED leaders can also promote pathway use by engaging local stakeholders to adapt and incorporate pathways into institutional guidelines. This process helps ensure the pathway meets the expectations of all the clinicians that might treat a particular patient, helps reduce confusion and conflict, and establishes a shared local standard of care.[20]

SHARED DECISION MAKING

SDM is another tool to support choosing an alternative disposition to admission in cases of diagnostic uncertainty.[5] Although definitions vary, SDM is generally described as the process of engaging patients to make a health care decision in collaboration with their clinician. It also presumes the provision of evidence-based information in an accessible format combined with consideration of the patient's specific circumstances and concerns.[21] Studies of SDM suggest that patients' risk tolerance is often higher than that of physicians, and thus SDM may result in fewer admissions.[5] One randomized controlled trial (RCT) found that, when patients with low-risk chest pain were provided with a visual display of their clinician's pretest probability of acute coronary syndrome, they more frequently decided against admission and further cardiac testing, with equivalent outcomes and increased satisfaction.[22] A more recent RCT found that patients being considered for hospitalization in an observation unit for cardiac testing were more involved in the decision making and chose to go home 15% more often when they engaged in a structured SDM process, without an increase in major adverse cardiac events.[23]

The practice of SDM can be complex, and simply providing patients with evidence has been found insufficient in helping them to reach an informed decision. Instead, SDM implies a conversation that incorporates evidence; conveyance of uncertainty; and consideration of the patient's unique situation, goals, and preferences.[24] Physicians generally seem to support the concept of SDM,[25] although, in practice, it seems there are many obstacles to widespread adoption, including concerns about how to discuss cost, convey clinical uncertainty, and engage with patients of varying backgrounds.[26] There have been calls for development of better technologies to support effective SDM, as well as integration of SDM skills into medical education and continued research on how to best implement and evaluate this practice.[27–29]

THE OPTIONS FOR ALTERNATIVES TO ADMISSION FROM THE EMERGENCY DEPARTMENT: RAPID FOLLOW-UP CLINICS, OBSERVATION UNITS, AND HOME HOSPITAL PROGRAMS
Rapid Follow-up Clinics

EDs serve many patients who face challenges accessing outpatient medical services. Without the ability to correct this access problem, clinicians may admit patients for conditions that could otherwise be managed outside of the hospital.[30] As a result of hospital crowding, the United Kingdom has aggressively targeted diagnosis and treatment of so-called ambulatory care–sensitive conditions for diversion from the inpatient setting to rapid follow-up clinics.[31] US Health care reform has similarly tried to extend outpatient resources through accountable care organizations, increased insurance access, and implementation of financial incentives to coordinate care and reduce avoidable inpatient costs. However, even insured patients may have difficulty coordinating outpatient care in a timely fashion. Moreover, night and weekend care in the ED is often not amendable to coordination with outpatient clinicians.[5]

Access to rapid follow-up clinics following an ED visit has been shown to be a safe and often cost-effective substitution for inpatient admission for a variety of carefully selected conditions, such as pulmonary embolism,[32,33] febrile neutropenia,[34] and diverticulitis.[35,36] One recent study of an emergency department diabetes rapid-referral program in Boston, Massachusetts, found patients who presented to the ED with dysglycemia but who were not in hyperglycemic crisis could be effectively and safely managed through rapid referral to an outpatient diabetes clinic.[37] A key component of this program was the ability of the emergency physician to directly schedule the patient for an appointment, regardless of time of day of presentation, and to discharge the patient with a specific appointment time. Compared with historical controls, enrolled patients were more than 10% less likely to be hospitalized or return to the ED within the following year, had more than $5000 less in institutional health care expenditures, and achieved greater hemoglobin A1c reductions.[37] Transitional care clinics have also shown some promise in creating a venue for patients not already engaged in primary care, and 1 study showed patients that followed up in these clinics had fewer subsequent ED visits.[38] Similarly, creation of an outpatient quick diagnosis unit in Spain resulted in significant decreases of more than half of inpatient hospitalizations compared with historical controls[39] (**Box 1**).

Observation Units

Observation units offer an alternative to inpatient admission for ED patients for whom discharge home seems unsafe or logistically unavailable.[40] These units have expanded in number and scope over the past 40 years and, by 2016, 44.6% of US EDs had an observation unit.[41] **Table 1** includes examples of conditions that require diagnostics and/or therapies that can commonly be managed in an observation unit.

Effect of observation units on emergency department length of stay, boarding, and crowding

Some studies have investigated observation units as a way to reduce ED length of stay (LOS) and ED crowding. There is variable experience with the effect of a unit on ED LOS, with most reporting at least modest reductions in ED LOS after implementation. The organization and policies of the unit affect this impact. For instance, 1 study in Canada found that an observation unit that was built by taking beds away from the main ED resulted in slightly longer or equivalent LOS for those patients.[42] A recent small pilot study described reductions in ED LOS with a protocol to move patients with chest pain directly to an observation unit from triage after an initial clinician screening examination using a protocol based on the HEART score. However, these gains were limited by delays in transporting patients between the ED and the observation unit.[43]

In many hospitals, patients with behavioral health emergencies are a large contributor to ED crowding, given the lack of inpatient psychiatric beds and the resulting long LOS for these patients. One recent study found that creation of a dedicated psychiatric ED observation unit helped reduce ED LOS to less than a quarter of what it was before intervention.[44] It also resulted in lower inpatient psychiatric admission rates, suggesting that investment in upfront full evaluation and treatment may reduce unnecessary use of scarce inpatient psychiatric beds.[44] Increasingly, EDs can now bill for observation services for psychiatric patients with extended stays, which may help in the development of best practices and protocols for this population.[45]

Box 1
Key points for successful use emergency department outpatient follow-up clinics as alternatives to admission

Create processes to allow direct outpatient clinic follow-up scheduling from the ED, regardless of time of day or day of week, in order to have patients leave with a specific appointment date and time in hand

Link follow-up clinic systems to use of a clinical diagnostic pathway that is accepted by both the referring ED and accepting specialty clinic

Table 1
Common observation conditions

Diagnostic Observation	Therapeutic Observation
Abdominal pain	Allergic reaction
Back pain	Asthma/COPD
Chest pain	Atrial fibrillation
Gastrointestinal bleed	Congestive heart failure
Mild traumatic brain injury	Dehydration/electrolyte abnormality
Nephrolithiasis	Dysglycemia
Psychiatric emergency	Headache
Neurologic complaint (TIA symptoms or seizure)	Infections: cellulitis, pneumonia, pyelonephritis
Syncope	Pulmonary embolism
Trauma	Transfusion

Abbreviations: COPD, chronic obstructive pulmonary disease; TIA, transient ischemic attack.

Observation units can also serve as a setting to perform expedited work-up and placement of patients who need postdischarge rehabilitation but who do not have a medical condition requiring inpatient admission. Observation units are an ideal setting for physical therapy assessments and engagement of case management. The Affordable Care Act's provision for an SNF waiver can facilitate rapid placement of patients requiring postdischarge rehabilitation care while avoiding the traditional 3-night inpatient Medicare requirement for coverage of the rehabilitation stay. A recent study of the Medicare Shared Savings Program reported cost savings among hospitals that used this program.[46] It is hoped that further expansion of the SNF waiver program will help support this workflow.

Definitions and evidence of value

Observation unit care has been shown to be significantly higher value than care of observation status patients in inpatient areas without protocolized care.[47] Studies have shown that observation units deliver equivalent outcomes with reduced hospital LOS for a variety of conditions, including heart failure,[48] transient ischemic attacks,[49,50] syncope,[40,41] and new-onset atrial fibrillation.[51] A systematic review of 139 studies of observation units found that advantages were shown in every study.[52] A recent Cochrane Review of available trials of short-stay units, encompassing observation units, also suggests that these units produce cost and time savings as well as improved patient satisfaction.[53]

Care delivered in an observation unit and care that is under the observation status are related but not the same. Observation is a billing status defined by the Centers for Medicare and Medicaid Services (CMS) as care used to determine whether inpatient admission is indicated that should span less than 2 midnights. Observation can and does therefore take place in any part of the hospital.[40] In contrast, observation care in an observation unit implies cohorting of patients within 1 location and treatment according to specific protocols, guidelines, and administrative processes. Units generally aim to serve patients with an 80% chance of discharge within the time frame outlined by CMS and a diagnostic or therapeutic question that is amenable to evidence-based protocolized care.[40,54] Patients treated within an observation unit usually, but not always, come under an observation billing status if cared for elsewhere in the hospital.

Observation best practices

A well-run observation unit with clear protocols and good administrative oversight has been shown to be most effective in delivering high-value care.[40,55] Many of the advantages stem from the shorter length of hospitalization achieved in these units compared with care provided in inpatient areas of the hospital. Best practices to support these time efficiencies include agreements with hospital leadership to prioritize observation patients for testing and consultations. This prioritization can be challenging for community practices, where consultants often have other responsibilities during the workday and may not have the flexibility to see a patient within a rapid time frame. Other strategies include encouraging disposition of patients on work-up completion, regardless of time of day.

Best practices also include choosing the right type of patient for a given observation unit. Not all observation units can manage all patients classified as observation, and some patients who are in observation status may be better served by an inpatient admission. For instance, although there is growing evidence that observation units can provide high-quality, efficient, and safe care for elderly and psychiatric patients, care of these special populations necessitates resources that are not available in every observation unit. When an observation unit first opens, it is typical to focus on a narrow set of conditions best supported by the literature as amenable to observation care (eg, chest pain, dehydration). Over time, as the staff gain experience and confidence with their observation capabilities, more challenging diagnoses (eg, congestive heart failure) are added to attempt to capture the maximum opportunity for cohorting the hospital's observation patients into 1 unit.

In contrast, observation units can provide high-value care to patients who might otherwise meet inpatient criteria because of intensity of treatment but are not expected to stay in the hospital more than 2 days.[40] Analysis of the 2007 National Hospital Ambulatory Medical Care Survey (NHAMCS) showed that patients who were inpatients for fewer than 2 days shared similar characteristics to observation patients and represented a possible area for expansion of these units.[56] An analysis of 2010 NHAMCS data predicted that, nationally, 11.7% of short-stay patients could be treated in a dedicated observation unit with a savings of up to $8.5 billion annually.[47] Placement of short-stay patients into observation units likely makes more sense at institutions that can backfill those inpatient beds with patients that have more complex needs or in institutions that are facing an ED crowding crisis.[40]

Ownership of the observation unit is another important consideration. Most observation units are run by the ED staff and accept only patients that originate from the ED. Some clinicians have argued that a more centralized model that accepts postsurgical and other types of patients may also be feasible and offer even greater cost and time efficiencies.[57] Others worry that opening units up to a variety of clinicians would create confusion, cause deviation from protocolized care, and result in inefficiencies.[40] Success of either model requires coordination among services and agreement on clear protocols.

Possible concerns and pitfalls of observation units

Despite their proven value, observation units can still be prone to misuse, and some clinicians warn that they can promote and protect sloppy decision making. One interview-based study with physicians in the United Kingdom and United States found that many clinicians view the observation unit as a safe space, where decisions made for medicolegal concerns, social problems, or decision fatigue can be hidden from and thus unchallenged by the rest of the hospital.[58] A study of emergency physician disposition decision making echoes this; the investigators concluded that the availability of an observation unit can support structured, evidence-based decision making, but it can also serve as a venue to avoid or delay making disposition decisions.[59] A related concern is that, given an observation unit, clinicians may choose to hospitalize patients that would otherwise have been appropriate for discharge, thus reducing the positive effects of observation units on patient LOS, costs, and hospital crowding. One study investigated patients with chest pain who were managed in an observation unit and predicted their disposition (admission or discharge) if that unit had not existed. Their model suggested that approximately half of those patients would have been discharged home had observation not been an option. However, their model could not determine whether observation was the safer or more efficient disposition for these patients.[60] This possible unintended consequence can likely be managed by creation of clear and protocolized observation pathways that include criteria for disposition home directly from the ED and a review process to catch and correct pitfalls of observation. Moreover, other studies have found that observation units can reduce admissions without also reducing discharges: 1 single-center before-and-after study of observation for acute exacerbations of chronic obstructive pulmonary disease found that inpatient admissions decreased 12% for this condition after implementation of an observation unit without affecting the proportion of patients directly discharged[61] (**Box 2**).

Home Hospital

Definitions and evidence base

Hospital at home programs offer another alternative to admission by shifting the location of care from the institution to the home for appropriate patients. There are many models for delivering acute care in the home, including home-based or office-based infusion programs and visiting nurse and physical therapist programs to promote early discharge, as well as more intensive home hospitalization programs.[62] There are 3 pathways to home hospital that can directly affect the ED and hospital capacity, collectively referred to as substitutive home hospital programs:

Emergency department substitution A community clinician refers the patient to the home hospital team in an effort to avoid a patient presenting to the ED. For example, a community clinician in the clinician's office may have diagnosed cellulitis in a patient that requires intravenous (IV) antibiotics. Instead of directing the patient to the ED or

---

Box 2
Key points for effective use of observation units as an alternative to inpatient admission

Encourage use of protocolized care through defined protocols and order sets. When possible, consider integrating these protocols into the electronic medical record.

Create systems that encourage clinicians to define clear goals and end points for the period of observation. Discourage use of observation for patients for whom another disposition is unclear or difficult, because of specialist push-back or incomplete work-up.

Consider carefully the scope of observation for the institution, which differs depending on resources and competing inpatient bed demands, including:
- Whether short-stay patients are well served in an observation unit
- Whether to accept more complex patients with anticipated longer observation duration (eg, >2 midnights)

Transport delays can minimize the gains an observation unit might provide with regard to decreasing ED LOS and ED crowding.

hospital, the community clinician can admit the patient to the home hospital team, who can then establish an IV, draw basic laboratory tests , and start IV antibiotics. This pathway saves both ED and hospital capacity.

Hospital substitution An emergency physician refers the patient to the home hospital team in an effort to avoid a hospitalization. For example, an emergency physician may have diagnosed a patient with pneumonia who requires hospitalization (eg, new oxygen requirement, need for IV therapies). Instead of hospitalizing the patient, the emergency physician can admit the patient to the home hospital team, who can then continue IV antibiotics, arrange oxygen as necessary, and reassess the patient's clinical status. This pathway saves hospital capacity and indirectly improves ED capacity by reducing boarding burden.

Inpatient length-of-stay substitution The admitting clinician refers the patient to the home hospital team to reduce the patient's hospital LOS. For example, a hospitalist may have stabilized a patient with congestive heart failure where the risk of decompensation has decreased, but the patient may require at least twice-a-day IV diuretics. Instead of continuing to hospitalize the patient for additional days, the hospitalist can transfer the care to the home hospital team, who can continue the IV diuretics, arrange to continue oxygen as necessary, and reassess the patient's clinical status. This pathway saves hospital and ED capacity by reducing the number of bed days used.

Substitutive home hospital programs have many reported benefits, including lower cost; increased patient satisfaction; lower rates of hospital-acquired infections, falls, and delirium; and a reduction in the need for continued institutional-based care such as rehabilitation after the hospitalization.[63–69] The home hospital concept has particular appeal for the care of elderly patients, for whom hospitalization has been shown to often cause harm through increased nosocomial infection, excessive noise, sensory deprivation, social isolation, and prolonged bed rest.[56–58]

Several RCTs have reported benefits of home hospital compared with inpatient care for a variety of conditions, including heart failure,[63] community-acquired pneumonia,[64] cellulitis,[65] and congestive obstructive pulmonary disease.[66,67] A 2009 meta-analysis of home hospital RCTs suggested significantly lower mortality at 6 months following discharge for home hospital patients; the reduction seen at 3 months was not statically significant.[68] A more recent Cochrane Review found that the home hospital strategy likely results in little or no difference in mortality outcomes but may increase the chance of the patient remaining at home following hospitalization and may result in greater patient satisfaction for appropriately selected patients and conditions.[69] Multiple studies have also shown significantly lower costs associated with the home hospital model.[66–68]

To date, most substitutive home hospital programs have been located in Canada, western Europe, New Zealand, and Australia, where, in Victoria, 2.5% of all inpatient admissions in 2008 were to a home hospital program.[70] There is much more limited experience in the United States. A nonrandomized study in Baltimore, Maryland, reported promising outcomes, with fewer complications such as delirium, higher patient and family satisfaction, and lower costs for patients treated at home compared with in a traditional acute hospital.[71] A small RCT of a pilot home hospital program in Boston, Massachusetts, found that patients had significantly more physical activity in the home hospital group and median costs were about half those of inpatient hospitalization. There was no detected difference in outcomes or satisfaction, although the small size of the pilot would make these differences difficult to detect.[72]

Organization of home hospital programs

Given the limited experience with substitutive home hospital programs in the United States, it is difficult to point out best practices in terms of organization, staffing, and protocols.

Home hospital programs incorporate 24-hour nurse and clinician coverage, with daily clinician visits and more frequent nursing visits. Patients within the programs have access to many of the services of the associated acute hospital, such as interpretation of imaging or video consultation with specialists.[71,72] Most use a hub-and-spoke model that enrolls patients within a defined catchment area close to the central facility, which limits the candidacy of otherwise-ideal patients for this program.

There are obvious challenges within this model to effective delivery of hospital-level care in the home. Although the ED operates 24 hours a day, the home hospital program may only be available to admit patients during certain hours. For example, a vendor may not be available after hours to deliver required durable medical equipment, such as oxygen. The outpatient pharmacy may also be unavailable after hours to provide an IV antibiotic for the patient's initial dose at home. The hub-and-spoke model creates obvious logistical challenges to expansion of services to a wider catchment area. Also, because of the need to travel from patient to patient, clinicians must navigate traffic, prioritize the order of rounding on patients, and maintain a flexible admission census. Technologies, such as remote telemetry and video visits, may help to mitigate these challenges. Also, there may also be opportunities to shift some of the in-home monitoring and service delivery to a mobile integrated health care model, using medical workers such as community paramedics who are already located closer to the patient's home.[73] Although this model has not yet been used in a US-based home hospital program, paramedics have been used successfully in other similar programs. For instance, New York City paramedics helped to treat approximately 2000 homebound individuals enrolled in an advanced illness management program, reducing use of the ED and inpatient setting to manage acute exacerbations.[74]

Like observation units, home hospital programs must choose their patients wisely. These programs may not be equipped to transport and still maintain care of patients that require advanced imaging such as MRI or invasive procedures such as cardiac catheterization. Furthermore, although patients are being monitored, rapid response to decompensation is limited and likely to require engagement of EMS, ideally using a mobile integrated health care model. These limitations require programs to have clearly defined admission criteria and robust screening processes to avoid a return to the acute hospital setting.

Clear payment structures have also yet to be defined, and this likely also limits home hospital expansion in the US health care market.[71] However, overall, home hospital programs seem to offer a viable alternative to traditional inpatient care by offering a

---

Box 3
Key points for effective use of home hospital programs as alternatives to inpatient admission

Choose patients wisely using clear inclusion and exclusion criteria.

Elderly patients may experience more harms than others in an institutional hospital setting and may be particularly well served by a home hospital program.

There are challenges to expanding the catchment area of programs. Exploring alternative staffing models, such as the use of a mobile integrated health care model and paramedics for some of the care delivered, may help address these.

setting that may be a more scalable and less costly alternative to building more hospital beds to safely provide care to patients with acute illness requiring an inpatient level of care (**Box 3**).

SUMMARY

Hospital crowding continues to compromise the ability of EDs to deliver safe and effective care to their patients. Alternatives to inpatient admission can help relieve crowding by providing another pathway out of the ED. Observation units and home hospital programs both offer alternatives to traditional inpatient admission. ADPs may be used alone or in conjunction with these dispositions to help support patients and clinicians in choosing a testing and treatment strategy that either avoids further work-up or relocates it to the less expensive and more efficient setting outside of the ED and hospital. In many cases, these alternatives also seem to be less costly and more efficient means to deliver equivalent quality of care compared with traditional inpatient admission. However, barriers of patient access, perceived medicolegal risk, and concerns over patient safety in the presence of diagnostic uncertainty will continue to pose challenges to widespread adoption of these strategies at some institutions.

DISCLOSURE

The authors have nothing to disclose.

REFERENCES

1. Singer AJ, Thode HC Jr, Viccellio P, et al. The association between length of emergency department boarding and mortality. Academic Emergency Medicine, vol. 18. John Wiley & Sons, Ltd (10.1111); 2011. p. 1324–9.
2. Gaieski DF, Agarwal AK, Mikkelsen ME, et al. The impact of ED crowding on early interventions and mortality in patients with severe sepsis. Am J Emerg Med 2017; 35:953–60.
3. Cha WC, Cho JS, Shin SD, et al. The impact of prolonged boarding of successfully resuscitated out-of-hospital cardiac arrest patients on survival-to-discharge rates. Resuscitation 2015;90:25–9.
4. Moskop JC, Geiderman JM, Marshall KD, et al. Another look at the persistent moral problem of emergency department crowding. Ann Emerg Med 2019;74: 357–64.
5. Schuur JD, Baugh CW, Hess EP, et al. Critical pathways for post-emergency outpatient diagnosis and treatment: tools to improve the value of emergency care. Acad Emerg Med 2011;18:e52–63.
6. Venkatesh AK, Dai Y, Ross JS, et al. Variation in US hospital emergency department admission rates by clinical condition. Med Care 2015;53:237–44.
7. Than M, Herbert M, Flaws D, et al. What is an acceptable risk of major adverse cardiac event in chest pain patients soon after discharge from the Emergency Department?: a clinical survey. Int J Cardiol 2013;166:752–4.
8. McCausland JB, Machi MS, Yealy DM. Emergency physicians' risk attitudes in acute decompensated heart failure patients. Acad Emerg Med 2010;17:108–10.
9. Van Den Berg P, Body R. The HEART score for early rule out of acute coronary syndromes in the emergency department: a systematic review and meta-analysis. Eur Heart J Acute Cardiovasc Care 2016;7:111–9.

10. Ò Miró, Peacock FW, McMurray JJ, et al. European Society of Cardiology – Acute Cardiovascular Care Association position paper on safe discharge of acute heart failure patients from the emergency department. Eur Heart J Acute Cardiovasc Care 2016;6:311–20.

11. Lindor RA, Boie ET, Campbell RL, et al. Failure to obtain computed tomography imaging in head trauma: a review of relevant case Law. Jang T, editor. Acad Emerg Med 2015;22:1493–8.

12. Mahler SA, Riley RF, Hiestand BC, et al. The HEART Pathway randomized trial: identifying emergency department patients with acute chest pain for early discharge. Circ Cardiovasc Qual Outcomes 2015;8:195–203.

13. Asher E, Reuveni H, Shlomo N, et al. Clinical outcomes and cost effectiveness of accelerated diagnostic protocol in a chest pain center compared with routine care of patients with chest pain. PLoS One 2015;10. e0117287–10.

14. Huis In 't Veld MA, Cullen L, Mahler SA, et al. The fast and the furious: low-risk chest pain and the rapid rule-out protocol. West J Emerg Med 2017;18:474–8.

15. Ljung L, Lindahl B, Eggers KM, et al. A rule-out strategy based on high-sensitivity troponin and HEART score reduces hospital admissions. Ann Emerg Med 2019; 73:491–9.

16. Fernando SM, Tran A, Cheng W, et al. Prognostic Accuracy of the HEART score for prediction of major adverse cardiac events in patients presenting with chest pain: a systematic review and meta-analysis. Acad Emerg Med 2019;26:140–51.

17. Yau AA, Nguyendo LT, Lockett LL, et al. The HEART pathway and hospital cost savings. Crit Pathw Cardiol 2017;16:126–8.

18. Dayan PS, Ballard DW, Tham E, et al. Use of traumatic brain injury prediction rules with clinical decision support. Pediatrics 2017;139:e20162709.

19. Vinson DR, Mark DG, Chettipally UK, et al. Increasing safe outpatient management of emergency department patients with pulmonary embolism: a controlled pragmatic trial. Ann Intern Med 2018;169:855–65.

20. Baugh CW, Clark CL, Wilson JW, et al. Creation and implementation of an outpatient pathway for atrial fibrillation in the emergency department Setting: Results of an Expert Panel. Hiestand BC, editor. Acad Emerg Med 2018;25:1065–75.

21. Makoul G, Clayman ML. An integrative model of shared decision making in medical encounters. Patient Educ Couns 2006;60:301–12.

22. Kline JA, Zeitouni RA, Hernandez-Nino J, et al. Randomized trial of computerized quantitative pretest probability in low-risk chest pain patients: effect on safety and resource use. Ann Emerg Med 2009;53:727–35.e1.

23. Hess EP, Hollander JE, Schaffer JT, et al. Shared decision making in patients with low risk chest pain: prospective randomized pragmatic trial. BMJ 2016;355: i6165.

24. Hargraves I, Leblanc A, Shah ND, et al. Shared decision making: the need for patient-clinician conversation, Not Just Information. Health Aff (Millwood) 2016; 35:627–9.

25. Kanzaria HK, Brook RH, Probst MA, et al. Emergency physician perceptions of shared decision-making. Acad Emerg Med 2015;22:399–405.

26. Zeuner R, Frosch DL, Kuzemchak MD, et al. Physicians' perceptions of shared decision-making behaviours: a qualitative study demonstrating the continued chasm between aspirations and clinical practice. Health Expect 2015;18: 2465–76.

27. Agoritsas T, Heen AF, Brandt L, et al. Decision aids that really promote shared decision making: the pace quickens. BMJ 2015;350:g7624.

28. Elwyn G, Frosch DL, Kobrin S. Implementing shared decision-making: consider all the consequences. Implement Sci Biomed Cent 2015;11:1–10.
29. Hess EP, Grudzen CR, Thomson R, et al. Shared decision-making in the emergency department: respecting patient autonomy when seconds count. Acad Emerg Med 2015;22:856–64.
30. Hunter AEL, Spatz ES, Bernstein SL, et al. Factors Influencing Hospital Admission of Non-critically Ill Patients Presenting to the Emergency Department: a Cross-sectional Study. J Gen Intern Med 2015;31:37–44.
31. Hamad MMAA, Connolly VM. Ambulatory emergency care - improvement by design. Clin Med 2018;18:69–74.
32. Zondag W, Exter den PL, Crobach MJT, et al. Comparison of two methods for selection of out of hospital treatment in patients with acute pulmonary embolism. Thromb Haemost 2017;109:47–52.
33. Piran S, Le Gal G, Wells PS, et al. Outpatient treatment of symptomatic pulmonary embolism: A systematic review and meta-analysis. Thromb Res 2013;132:515–9.
34. Mamtani M, Conlon LW. Can we safely discharge low-risk patients with febrile neutropenia from the emergency department? Ann Emerg Med 2014;63:48–51.
35. Jackson JD, Hammond T. Systematic review: outpatient management of acute uncomplicated diverticulitis. Int J Colorectal Dis 2014;29:775–81.
36. Conley J, O'Brien CW, Leff BA, et al. Alternative strategies to inpatient hospitalization for acute medical conditions: a systematic review. JAMA Intern Med 2016; 176:1693–702.
37. Palermo NE, Modzelewski KL, Farwell AP, et al. Open access to diabetes center from the emergency department reduces hospitalizations in the susequent year. Endocr Pract 2016;22:1161–9.
38. Elliott K, W Klein J, Basu A, et al. Transitional care clinics for follow-up and primary care linkage for patients discharged from the ED. Am J Emerg Med 2016;34:1230–5.
39. Bosch X, Jordán A, López-Soto A. Quick diagnosis units: avoiding referrals from primary care to the ED and hospitalizations. Am J Emerg Med 2013;31:114–23.
40. Mace SE. Observation Medicine: Principles and Protocols. 2017.
41. Rui P, Kang K, Ashman JJ. National Hospital Ambulatory Medical Care Survey: 2016 emergency department summary tables. 2016. Available at: https://www.cdc.gov/nchs/data/ahcd/nhamcs_emergency/2016_ed_web_tables.pdf
42. Cheng AHY, Barclay NG, Abu-Laban RB. Effect of a multi-diagnosis observation unit on emergency department length of stay and inpatient admission rate at two canadian hospitals. J Emerg Med 2016;51:739–47.e3.
43. Williams J, Aurora T, Baker K, et al. Triage to observation: a quality improvement initiative for chest pain patients presenting to the emergency department. Crit Pathw Cardiol 2019;18:75–9.
44. Parwani V, Tinloy B, Ulrich A, et al. Opening of psychiatric observation unit eases boarding crisis. Acad Emerg Med 2018;25:456–60.
45. McKenzie D, Granovsky M. Extended ED mental health care now reportable as observation. Dallas Texas: ACEP Now. American College of Emergency Physicians; 2019.
46. OEI HOOIG. ACOs' Strategies for Transitioning to Value-Based Care: Lessons From the Medicare Shared Savings Program (OEI-02-15-00451; 07/19). 2019 Jul pp. 1–44.
47. Ross MA, Hockenberry JM, Mutter R, et al. Protocol-driven emergency department observation units offer savings, shorter stays, and reduced admissions. Health Aff 2013;32:2149–56.

48. Schrager J, Wheatley M, Georgiopoulou V, et al. Favorable bed utilization and re-admission rates for emergency department observation unit heart failure patients. Acad Emerg Med 2013;20:554–61.

49. Jarhult S, Howell M, Barnaure-Nachbar I, et al. Implementation of a rapid, protocol-based TIA management pathway. West J Emerg Med 2018;19:216–23.

50. Stead LG, Bellolio MF, Suravaram S, et al. Evaluation of transient ischemic attack in an emergency department observation unit. neurocrit care, vol. 10. Humana Press Inc; 2008. p. 204–8.

51. Decker WW, Smars PA, Vaidyanathan L, et al. A prospective, randomized trial of an emergency department observation unit for acute onset atrial fibrillation. Ann Emerg Med 2008;52:322–8.

52. Baugh CW, Mace SE, and MPMP, 2017. The Evidence Basis for Observation Medicine in Adults Based on Diagnosis/Clinical Condition. Observation Medicine: Principles and Protocols. books.google.com; 2017.

53. Strøm C, Stefansson JS, Fabritius ML, et al. Hospitalisation in short-stay units for adults with internal medicine diseases and conditions. Cochrane Effective Practice and Organisation of Care Group. Cochrane Database Syst Rev 2018;(8):CD012370.

54. Ross MA, Granovsky M. History, principles, and policies of observation medicine. Emerg Med Clin 2017;35:503–18.

55. Conley J, Bohan JS, Baugh CW. The establishment and management of an observation unit. Emerg Med Clin 2017;35:519–33.

56. Wiler JL, Ross MA, Ginde AA. National study of emergency department observation services. Acad Emerg Med 2011;18:959–65.

57. Shah S, Subbarao K, Noonan MD, Hinrichs B. A new look at observation units: evidence-based approach. JHA 2015;5(6):115. https://doi.org/10.5430/jha.v4n6p115.

58. Martin GP, Wright B, Ahmed A, et al. Use or abuse? A qualitative study of physicians' views on use of observation stays at three hospitals in the United States and England. Ann Emerg Med 2016;69:284–92.e2.

59. Wright B, Martin GP, Ahmed A, et al. How the availability of observation status affects emergency physician decisionmaking. Ann Emerg Med 2018;72:401–9.

60. Blecker S, Gavin NP, Park H, et al. Observation units as substitutes for hospitalization or home discharge. Ann Emerg Med 2016;67:706–13.e2.

61. Budde J, Agarwal P, Mazumdar M, et al. Can an emergency department observation unit reduce hospital admissions for COPD exacerbation? Lung 2018;196:267–70.

62. Leff B. Defining and disseminating the hospital-at-home model. CMAJ 2009;180:156–7.

63. Tibaldi V, Isaia G, Scarafiotti C, et al. Hospital at home for elderly patients with acute decompensation of chronic heart failure: a prospective randomized controlled trial. Arch Intern Med 2009;169:1569–75.

64. Richards DA, Les J Toop, Epton MJ, et al. Home management of mild to moderately severe community-acquired pneumonia: a randomised controlled trial. Med J Aust 2005;183:235–8.

65. Corwin P, Toop LES, McGeoch G, et al. Randomised controlled trial of intravenous antibiotic treatment for cellulitis at home compared with hospital. BMJ 2005;330:129.

66. Nicholson C, Bowler S, Jackson C, et al. Cost comparison of hospital- and home-based treatment models for acute chronic obstructive pulmonary disease. Aust Health Rev 2001;24:181–7.

67. Davies L, Wilkinson M, Bonner S, et al. "Hospital at home" versus hospital care in patients with exacerbations of chronic obstructive pulmonary disease: prospective randomised controlled trial. BMJ 2000;321:1265–8.
68. Shepperd S, Doll H, Angus RM, et al. Avoiding hospital admission through provision of hospital care at home: a systematic review and meta-analysis of individual patient data. CMAJ 2009;180:175–82.
69. Shepperd S, Iliffe S, Doll HA, et al. Admission avoidance hospital at home. Cochrane Effective Practice and Organisation of Care Group. Cochrane Database Syst Rev 2016;10:S29–67.
70. Montalto M. The 500-bed hospital that isn't there: the Victorian Department of Health review of the Hospital in the Home program. Med J Aust 2010;193:598–601.
71. Leff B, Burton L, Mader SL, et al. Hospital at home: feasibility and outcomes of a program to provide hospital-level care at home for acutely ill older patients. Ann Intern Med 2005;143:798–808.
72. Levine DM, Ouchi K, Blanchfield B, et al. Hospital-level care at home for acutely ill adults: a pilot randomized controlled trial. J Gen Intern Med 2018;33:729–36.
73. Vision Statement on Mobile Integrated Healthcare (MIH) & Community Paramedicine (CP). 2015 Mar pp. 1–3.
74. Abrashkin KA, Poku A, Ramjit A, et al. Community paramedics treat high acuity conditions in the home: a prospective observational study. BMJ Support Palliat Care 2019. https://doi.org/10.1136/bmjspcare-2018-001746.

Quality Assurance in the Emergency Department

William E. Baker, MD[a], Joshua J. Solano, MD[b],*

KEYWORDS

- Clinical competence • Emergency department • Emergency medicine • Peer review
- Health care • Quality of health care • Quality assurance

KEY POINTS

- Quality assurance of health care involves activities aimed at ensuring that the care provided meets applicable standards.
- Health care delivery is complex, and a wide range of factors affect quality of care; quantification of health care quality is challenging in large part due to this complexity.
- Determination of deviation from acceptable care (and justification of such deviation if applicable) is integral to quality reviews.
- Practitioner competency evaluation is one component of quality assurance, and emergency medicine (EM) physicians should be familiar with that process, particularly (for US EM physicians) the framework defined by the Center for Medicare and Medicaid Services.
- Peer review of cases derived either from direct referral or via triggers remains a fundamental component of an overall quality assurance program.

INTRODUCTION

At the beginning of the twentieth century, Ernest Amory Codman advocated for the "End Result Idea" that hospitals follow their patients longitudinally to see the effects of their treatment and outcomes, which was revolutionary at the time.[1,2] His pioneering work in clinical medicine and quality improvement helped lead to the creation of the Joint Commission on Accreditation of Hospitals to help standardize hospitals (JCAHO), later changing names simply to the Joint Commission (JC). Emergency department (ED) quality assurance (QA) has its historical underpinnings in Joint Commission's mandate to monitor QA in hospital-based EDs.[3] This broad mandate encompassed the clinical care environment, operational and systems issues, and

[a] Department of Emergency Medicine, Boston University, Boston University Medical Center, 800 Harrison Avenue, Boston, MA 02118, USA; [b] Integrated Medical Science, Florida Atlantic University, Boca Raton, FL, USA
* Corresponding author. Department of Emergency Medicine, Bethesda Hospital East, 2815 South Seacrest Boulevard, Boynton Beach, FL 33435.
E-mail address: solanoj@health.fau.edu
Twitter: @EMDocBaker (W.E.B.); @JSolano_EM (J.J.S.)

Emerg Med Clin N Am 38 (2020) 663–680
https://doi.org/10.1016/j.emc.2020.05.002
0733-8627/20/© 2020 Elsevier Inc. All rights reserved.

emed.theclinics.com

physician competency. After the Institute of Medicine (IOM) published *To Err is Human*, the ED was implicated as one "hospital location with the highest proportion of negligent adverse events."[4] This, along with the patient safety and quality improvement movement across medicine, has led stakeholders to focus QA in EDs (**Box 1**). In 2016, American EDs managed 145 million visits, 12.6 million hospitalizations, and 2.2 million admissions to an intensive care unit.[5] Despite the vast effort devoted to improve the quality of care in EDs, publicly reported quality data only captures timing measures such as ED length of stay and specific conditions such as acute myocardial infarction management.[6]

GENERAL QUALITY ASSURANCE OVERVIEW

QA involves a set of activities that monitor a product or service provided, providing confidence that it fulfills its requirements for quality. A cornerstone of QA within medicine is agreement on definitions of the quality of care. In 1990, an IOM study committee addressed this topic through examining key dimensions used to define quality. They settled on 18 dimensions, a select few being the following:

- A scale of quality, nature of entity being evaluated
- Type of recipient identified (individual, population, patient type)
- Technical competency of providers
- Interpersonal skills of practitioners
- Standards of care

The IOM concluded that "...quality of care is the degree to which health services for individuals and populations increase the likelihood of desired health outcomes and are consistent with current professional knowledge."[7]

In another landmark work, *Crossing the Quality Chasm: A New Health System for the 21st Century,* the IOM described what is now one of the most influential frameworks for quality assessment. The following are their 6 specific aims of quality, which the

---

Box 1
Organizations involved in quality assurance in the emergency departments in the United States

American Board of Emergency Medicine (ABEM)

American College of Emergency Physicians (ACEP)

Centers for Medicare and Medicaid Services (CMS)

Accreditation Council for Graduate Medical Education (ACGME) via the Clinical Learning Environment Review (CLER)

Emergency Department Benchmarking Alliance

The Leapfrog Group

Joint Commission on Accreditation of Healthcare Organizations

Agency for Healthcare Research and Quality

National Quality Forum

Institute for Healthcare Improvement

Society for Academic Emergency Medicine

US Department of Health and Human Services

Agency for Healthcare Research and Quality (AHRQ) has adopted as the "Six Domains of Health Care Quality":

1. Safe—avoiding injuries to patients from the care that is intended to help them.
2. Effective—providing services based on scientific knowledge to all who could benefit and refraining from providing services to those not likely to benefit (avoiding underuse and overuse).
3. Patient-centered—providing care that is respectful of and responsive to individual patient preferences, needs, and values and ensuring that patient values guide all clinical decisions.
4. Timely—reducing waits and sometimes harmful delays for both those who receive and those who give care.
5. Efficient—avoiding waste, in particular waste of equipment, supplies, ideas, and energy.
6. Equitable—providing care that does not vary in quality because of personal characteristics such as gender, ethnicity, geographic location, and socioeconomic status.[8,9]

Medical errors (MEs) and adverse events (AEs) define a major area of focus for ED QA. The report *To Err is Human: Building a Safer Health System* defines an error as "the failure of a planned action to be completed as intended (ie, error of execution) or the use of a wrong plan to achieve an aim (ie, error of planning). An AE is an injury caused by medical management rather than the underlying condition of the patient. An AE attributable to error is a "preventable AE." Negligent AEs represent a subset of preventable AEs that satisfy legal criteria used in determining negligence (ie, whether the care provided failed to meet the standard of care reasonably expected of an average physician qualified to take care of the patient in question)."[4,10] These definitions help focus on systems of care as well as individuals.

Currently, the 3 aims of the National Quality Strategy (NQS) defined in 2011 from the Agency for Healthcare Research and Quality are

1. Better care
2. Healthy people and communities
3. Affordable care[11]

In order to advance these aims, the NQS outlines the following priorities:

- Making care safer by reducing harm caused in the delivery of care
- Ensuring that each person and family is engaged as partners in their care
- Promoting effective communication and coordination of care
- Promoting the most effective prevention and treatment practices for the leading causes of mortality, starting with cardiovascular disease
- Working with communities to promote wide use of best practices to enable healthy living
- Making quality care more affordable for individuals, families, employers, and governments by developing and spreading new health care delivery models.

EMERGENCY DEPARTMENT QUALITY ASSURANCE OVERVIEW

The ED is critical to accomplishing the 3 aims. Each of the priorities can be summarized as patient safety, timeliness, effectiveness, equity of care, patient-centeredness, and the reduction of MEs and AEs.[8] The ED, in the United States, has a major role in most communities by providing access for the acute needs for those who are ill or injured. It serves as a safety net with 24 hours a day/7 days a week access to emergency medical care irrespective of the ability to pay due to the Emergency Medicine Treatment and Labor Act.[12,13]

ED QA's original focus to identify MEs and AEs through retrospective review of cases has yielded many of the current processes of QA, used by many EDs throughout the United States.[3,14–16] Popular strategies have included systemic reviews of deaths in the ED, 72-hour returns, patient complaints, and other triggers noted in **Box 2**.[17–20] Recent studies have criticized these measures as low-yield for identifying MEs and AEs,[21] yet they may miss approximately 90% of the AEs.[22]

Academic emergency medicine departments have a mandate from the Accreditation Council for Graduate Medical Education (ACGME) to include quality improvement activities, morbidity and mortality conferences, and patient safety as part of residency training.[23] This requirement has led to the development of more robust, resource-intensive, and complicated systems at academic medical center EDs.[21] In community EDs, QA is often conducted by an ED director or assistant director and may focus only on complaints ("problem" cases specifically referred for review) in a department or the publicly reported measures. The rest of the QA may be instituted at the departmental level or nursing administration, with the publicly reported mandates being reported at the hospital level.

EMERGENCY DEPARTMENT QUALITY COMMITTEE

The structure of a quality committee for the ED is multidisciplinary and has been described by Klasco and colleagues[17] to include physicians, nurses, hospital QA representation, and ancillary staff. This committee receives input from screened cases by trigger processes developed by the department or the hospital. The QA can then refer cases to different parties within the hospital. A diagram of this structure is included in **Fig. 1**. Typically, more parties are involved at academic then community centers. Membership in this committee may rotate and this can be used with mentorship for residents or junior attendings to become involved in the QA processes. A model from the hospital's peer review committee may be used with a term of membership, scheduled meetings, and involvement of stakeholders.

MEASUREMENTS AND METRICS IN THE EMERGENCY DEPARTMENT

The EDs QA measures have focused on several pathologic conditions that entail significant morbidity and mortality and have well-defined standards of care or adopted

---

Box 2
Commonly used emergency department quality assurance triggers

Deaths in the ED (within specified time period)

72-hour returns (with and without admission)

Patient complaints

Internal referrals

Physician complaints/nursing complaints (external referrals)

Floor-to-ICU transfers (upgrades in care)

Procedural sedation

Review of certain pathologic conditions (ie, Sepsis, Stroke, STEMI)

Transfer to other facilities

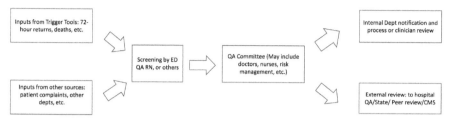

Fig. 1. ED QA process structure. (*Adapted from* Klasco RS, Wolfe RE, Wong M, et al. Assessing the Rates of Error and Adverse Events in the ED. Am J Emerg Med. 2015 Dec;33(12):1786-9; with permission.)

guidelines. Notable examples include acute stroke and ST-elevation myocardial infarction (STEMI). Door-to-balloon time for STEMI and related process measures were originally created by the American College of Cardiology in conjunction with the American Heart Association and involve the coordination of EDs, emergency medical services, and catheterization laboratory teams.[24] This metric was developed in 2006 and its effects have been transformative. The ED is a crucial part of the process, and delays within the ED remain an area of active improvement.[25] In the parlance of QA, *measures* refer to processes that can be measured, whereas *metrics* define a goal for a measured process. For instance, originally door-to-balloon time was measured, and the optimal time of 90 minutes was defined as a metric to meet or exceed for patients with an STEMI (inclusive of a door-to-electrocardiogram time goal <10 minutes).[26] Eventually, metrics may be adjusted or systems may define their own metrics from commonly measured processes.

The defining of metrics and their link to payment presents dangers and opportunities for EDs and emergency physicians. Historically many metrics have been established with minimal participation of the emergency medicine community. Two such examples include the time to initiate antibiotics (within 4 hours of arrival) for community-acquired pneumonia and obtaining blood cultures before the administration of antibiotics.[27] Both recommendations were eventually removed but not before there was widespread criticism that the recommendations were not evidence based and were potentially harmful to patients.

EMERGENCY DEPARTMENT QUALITY ASSURANCE PAYMENT AND SYSTEMS FOR REPORTING

The emphasis on measuring the quality of care has led to more disease-defined metrics. Multiple organizations have released ED quality markers (see **Box 1**)[28]—some attributable to individual providers but many related to systems and the clinical care environment. The Patient Protection and Affordable Care Act in 2010 tied some of these measures into the Quality Payment Program (QPP) most commonly through the Merit-based Incentive Payment System (MIPS).[29] These programs help replace CMS's voluntary physician quality reporting system to report, measure, and reward physician quality.[30] Under the current system, hospitals, clinicians, and groups must report metrics or face penalties and reduced reimbursement.[31]

Clinical Emergency Data Registry is an EM specialty-wide registry supported by the American College of Emergency Physicians (ACEP) designed to measure EM outcomes, identify practice patterns, improve quality of acute care, and meet QPP/MIPS quality reporting for those not in the alternative payment model.[32] The registry now contains about 250 practice groups, more than 1000 individual EDs, and accounts for 25 million ED visits.[33] Its goal is to create new measures and apply big data analytics to improve patient care. The Emergency Quality Network is another quality collaborative sponsored through ACEP,[34] currently focused on improving quality of care for sepsis, imaging, chest pain, and opioid management.[34]

PITFALLS IN MEASUREMENTS

Future QA measures could revolve around chief complaints,[35] for instance, whether or not a female patient of child-bearing age with abdominal pain receives pregnancy testing. However, even a simple measure such as this can be fraught with error. The measure might be determined by a specific pregnancy test recorded in a single field of the medical record. If this is the preferred indicator, other methods to rule out pregnancy, such as the use of a bedside pregnancy test, surgical status such as hysterectomy, or outside records could unwittingly fail the measure.[36] If physicians then learn they will fail the process measure without a specific test, they may do this just to "meet the measure" and overutilize resources.

Gaps in Emergency Department Quality Assurance

Other issues with QA include incomplete measurement of diagnostic errors, limited outpatient follow-up, and transitions of care. Care can be efficient, fast, and wrong, yet still be rated well by time measures. Because patients do not always present back to the same provider or system, diagnostic errors may elude the first institution. A patient with an obstructing kidney stone who did not have urine collected (visit lasted less than 2 hours) could go to another institution in septic shock. A patient who presents with a cough and has a chest radiograph within an hour may pass a timeliness metric, but if the radiograph shows a pulmonary nodule, and the need for follow-up is not communicated, the patient's preventable cancer could be missed. The current system of time-based fee-for-service productivity would reward both visits despite the clear MEs and AEs.

Efforts to reduce utilization or overtesting have also been difficult to implement. Concerns about limiting clinician decision-making and increasing diagnostic errors are weighed against overutilization.[37] Ultimately, reducing variation and improving the use of evidence-based medicine requires careful attention to what is being measured and how it affects clinicians, systems, and patients. Numerous attempts to game the system are seen in assigning EM service codes,[38] and high-stake measures may experience a Hawthorne effect until their metrics are retired.

Systems-level issues compound these existing challenges. The siloing of information between different hospital systems creates major barriers in clinical care and makes comprehensive ED QA more difficult, as patients transfer between systems.[39] Likewise, the disparate measures that are currently used will likely expand, and payers are increasingly reducing payments to "low performers" and rewarding "top performers." Patient surveys of clinicians are also likely from the basis for further metrics, despite their historically checkered past and lack of validity.[40] Therefore, as more reimbursement is tied to QA metrics, clinicians and other stakeholders will need to selectively champion evidence-based metrics to ensure that they meaningfully improve patient care.

HOSPITAL-BASED PROVIDER PRIVILEGING AND COMPETENCY ASSESSMENT

The Centers for Medicare and Medicaid Services (CMS) is the single largest payer of health care services in the United States and as such, the CMS is highly influential in setting health care standards. Hospitals participating in the Medicare program must adhere to a set of requirements for privileging and competency assessment pertaining to their medical staff. These requirements include an appraisal of every individual medical staff member's qualifications for each privilege, as well as a system for demonstrating competency in those privileges granted every 24 months or earlier (irrespective of board certification).[41] Hospital participation in the CMS program requires accreditation, either directly from CMS or through a CMS-approved program. This process involves regular surveys to certify compliance with the Medicare requirements.[42] The Joint Commission (JC) is the most widely used CMS-approved accreditation program, accrediting 70% of the hospitals in the United States. Thus, JC requirements apply directly to most of the EM physicians in the United States.[43] CMS and JC requirements are predominantly interchangeable, with JC standards being referenced more specifically.

Among JC-accredited hospitals, physicians (and other medical practitioners) are organized into a self-governing body termed "the medical staff" that oversees the quality of care provided by all members privileged at the organization. Toward that goal, the medical staff is required to evaluate staff members' privilege-specific competency and behavior through the frameworks of "Focused Professional Practice Evaluation" (FPPE) and "Ongoing Professional Practice Evaluation" (OPPE).[42] The JC has integrated into its competency requirements the same 6 core competencies (practice-based learning and improvement, patient care and procedural skills, systems-based practice, medical knowledge, interpersonal and communication skills, and professionalism) used by the ACGME and the American Board of Medical Specialties (ABMS).[23,44,45]

FPPE is performed for all initial privileges granted at a specific organization, the most common scenario being a newly appointed hospital staff member (or ED hire).[44,46] Established, credentialed physicians granted new privileges at that hospital must also undergo FPPE. For instance, if a physician has been practicing at a hospital and then applies for and is granted a new privilege, they must undergo FPPE for that privilege (and OPPE for all existing privileges as per the scheduled review cycle). FPPE processes must be clearly defined by each hospital and must include the following 4 components:

1. Criteria for conducting performance monitoring
2. Method for establishing a monitoring plan specific to the requested privilege
3. Method for determining the duration of performance monitoring
4. Circumstances under which monitoring by an external source is required[44,47]

Although FPPE must be time limited, the JC defers to the organization to define the duration of monitoring and suggests considering monitoring numbers (ie, procedures or admissions) rather than duration in circumstances of a low volume privilege.[48]

Thereafter, OPPE is performed to assess competency for existing privileges and, per JC standards, is "A document summary of ongoing data collected for the purpose of assessing a practitioner's clinical competence and professional behavior. The information gathered during this process is factored into decisions to maintain, revise, or revoke existing privilege(s)..." for the purposes of consideration of privilege renewal at the end of the aforementioned 2-year cycle. Examples of data sources suggested by the JC include chart review, direct observation, monitoring of techniques, and discussion with others involved in the patient's care. Other data recommended for evaluation include compliance with JC Core Measures and patient readmissions (either inpatient or outpatient) for the same diagnosis or problem.[49] The JC have indicated a desire for monitoring that includes at least some measures involving a numerator and denominator, benchmarked against a standard, preferably national, at minimum compared with organizational peers. Such monitoring must occur more frequently than every 12 months. The JC suggests organizations consider an 8-month interval, providing 3 sets of data for the practitioner's 2-year renewal cycle.[44,46,50]

FPPE is also conducted for cause or when questions arise regarding a currently credentialed practitioner's competency. Triggers can be single incidents, such as a sentinel event or significant single complaint, or related to trends, such as (per the JC) "patterns of unnecessary diagnostic testing/treatments". Low volume alone over an extended time period can trigger an FPPE.

Choosing practitioner-relevant FPPE/OPPE measures is challenging. Systems and patient factors can influence results in most practitioners' competency measures. In addition, it can be difficult to prove that a particular measure is a true quality indicator of physician performance. One such example is the rate of unscheduled 72-hour return visits to the ED. This measure has its roots in the Maryland Hospital Association Quality Indicator Project (which began in 1985) and has been used for decades.[51] The AHRQ categorizes such a return visit as a "discharge failure" and the Institute for Healthcare improvement recommends that return visits with admission (48 hours) be a trigger for case reviews.[52,53] Controversy surrounds the utility of return visits as a quality indicator (including with respect to the timing of the return).[21,54-57] A recent study by Aaronson reviewing 413,167 ED visits identified that only 0.48% (n = 2001) of 72-hour returns were admitted to the hospital and only 2.49% (n = 50) of those involved deviation from optimal care. The investigators concluded that simply screening for 72-hour returns with admission has a low yield (<3%) for identifying suboptimal care. They did acknowledge that detailed case reviews can be useful for OPPE, as care deviation events most often represented errors in the diagnostic pathway.[58] Only a small body of peer-reviewed literature directly assesses the topic of FPPE/OPPE, and as of this review, only a single paper (by Walker and colleagues) addresses the implementation of FPPE/OPPE in emergency medicine. This study involved a current state survey, demonstrating considerable variation among respondents, with just greater than 65% using measures pertaining to "quality metrics," whereas 72-hour returns were used by 50% of respondents. Few regarded grading measures as "meaningful," whereas larger groups endorsed the measures as only "somewhat meaningful" or not useful. Further discussion with a subset of respondents noted that the majority were against measures such as ED length of stay for admitted patients and left without being seen rates, whereas peer review (of cases) was felt to be the most useful measure in judging provider competency.[59] So, 100 years after Codman's work, physicians choose peer review as a measure that is the best reflection of patient outcomes.

Perhaps one reason why physicians favor peer review of cases is that despite ACGME, ABMS, and CMS' focus on nontechnical core competencies such as professionalism and communication skills, there is little agreed-upon structure for their assessment. Furthermore, the 6 ACGME core competencies are not necessarily comprehensive in categorizing skills and behaviors. A comprehensive review out of the United Kingdom of nontechnical skills linked to safety and error in the ED identified a total of 34 skills and behaviors, condensed into 9 broad skills.[60]

Another facet of competency is perspective. The practice of emergency medicine involves considerable interprofessional collaboration, particularly with nurses. One study sought to identify nurses' views on EM physician competency, and the resultant model included aspects of the ACGME competencies but also emotional intelligence, problem-solving and decision-making skills, patient focus, operations management, and team leadership and management.[61]

Although work on a definition of appropriate EM competencies continues, practical ways of measuring them remain elusive. The same United Kingdom group referenced above developed an a non-technical skills assessment tool and includes a behavioral marker system (**Fig. 2**). Each assessment involves 1 hour of direct observation and assessment of each subject being evaluated, a cost that may prove too burdensome for EDs to bear.[62]

TAXONOMY OF EVENTS

The importance of a standardized terminology of AEs or incidents was championed by the IOM in their 2003 publication *Patient Safety: Achieving a New Standard of Care.*[63] There are many facets to such a taxonomy, the most basic and critical components are to define what constitutes an "incident," to categorize the level of harm associated with an incident, and to consider associated contributing patient and system factors. Several organizations have developed and promote particular patient safety taxonomy systems; however, consensus is lacking.

Since 2005, the World Health Organization's World Alliance for Patient Safety has undertaken the *Project to Develop an International Classification for Patient Safety* (ICPS) toward these goals and in 2009 published their conceptual framework, which involves the following:

- "Clinically meaningful" categories (incident type and patient outcomes)
- System resilience (detection, mitigating factors, and ameliorating actions)
- Descriptive information (contributing factors/hazards, patient and incident characteristics, and organizational outcomes)

They define a patient safety incident as "an event or circumstance that could have resulted, or did result, in unnecessary harm to a patient," more specifically labeled as a reportable circumstance, near miss, no harm incident, or harmful incident (AE).[64] JC also recognized the importance of standardizing taxonomy and in 2005 produced their own *Patient Safety Event Taxonomy* (**Fig. 3**), which the JC continues to reference.[65,66] The IHI uses a harm assessment tool adapted from the *National Coordinating Council for Medication Error Reporting and Prevention* (NCC MERP) Index for Categorizing Errors, derived in 1991 and recommends that it can be applied to nonmedication-related events (**Box 3**).[52,67] This taxonomy is available from the NCC MERP site along with supporting materials.[68] The AHRQ uses a harm assessment framework that grades degree and duration of harm (**Table 1**).[69] The American Society for Healthcare Risk Management has also adopted the AHRQ harm assessment framework and specifies that with respect to duration of harm, that "temporary" refers to harm with expected duration of less than 1 year and "permanent" means greater than 1 year.[70]

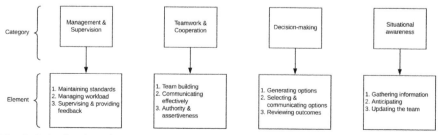

Fig. 2. Behavioral marker system. (*Adapted from* Flowerdew L, Brown R, Vincent C, et al. Development and Validation of a tool to Assess Emergency Physicians' Nontechnical Skills. Ann Emerg Med. 2012 May;59(5):376-385.e4; with permission.)

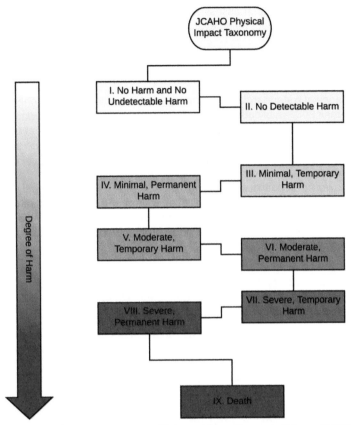

Fig. 3. JCAHO physical impact taxonomy. (*Adapted from* Chang A, Schyve JCAHO Medical, Physical Classification of Impact Taxonomy; with permission. And *Adapted from* Chang A, Schyve PM, Croteau RJ, et al. The JCAHO Patient Safety Event Taxonomy: A Standardized Terminology and Classification Schema for Near Misses and Adverse Events. Int J Qual Health Care J Int Soc Qual Health Care. 2005; 17(2):95-105; with permission.)

DEVIATION AND DETERMINATION OF QUALITY OF CARE AND CAUSATION

The concept of "deviation" in health care delivery is also critical but nuanced. Deviations occur when care does not adhere to a standard of care, which may include evidence-based or consensus guidelines, relevant policies or protocols, or a "reasonable person comparison"—what most of the clinician's peers might do in a similar circumstance.

However, deviation alone is not synonymous with harm or a lower quality of care. Deviations may be justifiable in particular situations. When harm to a patient has occurred, unjustified deviation serves as the basis for determining preventability. In assessing for deviation, it is also important to use a framework that considers factors of the surrounding system in which the deviation took place. Too often, focus is on "human error," fault and blame rather than a system analysis framework that considers all factors that may have contributed to an event.

One such framework is *The London Protocol*,[71] which is based on research outside of health care in aviation, oil and nuclear industries, and involves an "accident" investigational model. The accident causation model uses a "Framework of Contributory Factors Influencing Clinical Practice":

Box 3
Taxonomy of outcome

I. No Error
  a. Category A: circumstances or events that have the capacity to cause error

II. Error, No Harm
  a. Category B: error occurred but did not reach patient
  b. Category C: error occurred, reached patient, but did not cause harm
  c. Category D: error occurred reached the patient and required monitoring to confirm that it resulted in no harm to the patient, no intervention required

III. Error, Harm
  a. Category E: an error occurred that may have contributed to or resulted in temporary harm to the patient and required intervention
  b. Category F: an error occurred that may have contributed to or resulted in temporary harm to the patient and required initial or prolonged hospitalization
  c. Category G: an error occurred that may have contributed to or resulted in permanent patient harm
  d. Category H: an error occurred that required intervention necessary to sustain life

IV. Error, Death
  a. Category I: an error occurred that may have contributed to or resulted in the patient's death

Adapted from National Coordinating Council for Medication Error Reporting and Prevention. *NCC MERP Taxonomy of Medication Errors.* https://www.nccmerp.org/taxonomy-medication-errors-now-available 1998.

---

1. Patient factors
  a. Condition (complexity and severity)
  b. Language/communications
  c. Personality/social factors

Table 1
The agency for healthcare research and quality extent of harm

Death	Dead at Time of Assessment
Severe permanent harm	Severe permanent harm: severe lifelong bodily or psychological injury or disfigurement that interferes significantly with functional ability or quality of life
Permanent harm	Lifelong bodily or psychological injury or increased susceptibility to disease. Prognosis at time of assessment
Temporary harm	Bodily or psychological injury but likely not permanent
Additional treatment	Injury limited to additional intervention during admission or encounter and/or increased length of stay but no other injury. Treatment since discovery and/or expected treatment in future as a direct result of event
Emotional distress or inconvenience	Mild and transient anxiety or pain or physical discomfort but without the need for additional treatment other than monitoring (such as by observation; physical examination; laboratory testing, including phlebotomy; and/or imaging studies). Distress/inconvenience since discovery and/or expected in future as a direct result of event
No harm	Event reached patient, but no harm was evident
Unknown	

Adapted from Agency for Healthcare Research and Quality. *Extent of Harm.* U.S. Department of Health & Human Services; 2013.

2. Task and technology factors
   a. Task design and clarity of structure
   b. Availability and use of protocols
   c. Availability and accuracy of test results
   d. Decision-making aids
3. Individual (staff) factors
   a. Knowledge and skills
   b. Competence
   c. Physical and mental health
4. Team factors
   a. Verbal communications
   b. Written communications
   c. Supervision and seeking help
   d. Team structure
5. Work environmental factors
   a. Staffing levels and skills mix
   b. Workload and shift patterns
   c. Design, availability, and maintenance of equipment
   d. Administrative and managerial support
   e. Environment
   f. Physical
6. Organizational and management factors
   a. Financial resources and constraints
   b. Organizational structure
   c. Policy, standards, and goals
   d. Safety culture and priorities
7. Institutional context factors
   a. Economic and regulatory context
   b. Links with external organizations

For a more comprehensive understanding of "human error" or rather the role of systems factors in contributing to "human error," the reader is referred to *The Field Guide To Understanding 'Human Error', Third Edition.*[72]

QUALITY REVIEW STRATEGIES—CURRENT STATE, LIMITATIONS, AND FUTURE DIRECTIONS

An ideal QA process would involve manual review of all cases in which there was harm or deviation of care with the potential for harm, and only those cases, as well as mechanisms for monitoring the surrounding processes of care for deviation from acceptable standards. Unfortunately, this is an ideal state, rather than a feasible goal for many departments.

Current strategies of case review include identifying cases based on triggers and random auditing. Triggers for review may include individual referrals, such as the filing of patient safety events, or consensus-derived triggers (such as 72-hour return visits to the ED, transfers to higher level of care, or deaths). The yield of true AEs from this traditional surveillance-based strategy is low. It is essential that reviewers do not conflate crude rates of triggers with the prevalence of AEs or care defects. The IHI, in their *Global Trigger Tool for Measuring Adverse Events*, acknowledges the complexity of this topic, stating "…only 10 to 20 percent of errors are ever reported and, of those, 90 to 95 percent cause no harm to patients."[52] The ED module of the *Global Trigger Tool* includes only 2 triggers: return visits to the ED resulting in admission and ED length of stay greater than 6 hours, although some of their universal care triggers, such as transfusion of blood, restraints, falls, procedure complications, and transfer to higher level of care are applicable to ED patients.

Unplanned intensive care unit transfer (UIT) is another trigger of doubtful utility as an independent quality measure. The use of UITs involves multiple assumptions that have not been thoroughly validated. For instance, there is no standard determining the need for intensive care unit (ICU) level of care. Although cases involving acute initiation of mechanical ventilation or vasopressor therapy almost universally require ICU level of care, considerable practice variation exists for other reasons (such as "close monitoring"). In examining 108,732 non-ICU admissions from a single center's 520,202 ED visits, only 923 patients (0.9%) were identified as having either expired (n = 86) or were transferred (n = 837, 0.76%) to an ICU within 48 hours of initial ward admission. The investigators developed a list of 25 "critical interventions" (CrIs), which require ICU level of care. They excluded patients with active comfort-measures-only, do-not-resuscitate, or do-not-intubate orders on admission, postoperative complications, and planned ICU transfers. After applying these exclusion criteria, only 6% were judged to involve an ME, whereas 7% transfers that did not undergo a CrI involved an ME. Overall, for 108,732 patients admitted to a non-ICU setting, only 0.03% were transferred to an ICU within 48 hours and involved an ME. Although review of UIT with CrI may have some utility, crude rates of UIT are a poor measure of quality,[73] and its use as a performance marker may lead to over-utilization via "prophylactic" ICU care for patients. The use of more sophisticated, statistical approaches to identifying cases with AEs is a promising venue for improvement, but requires further research.[74]

SUMMARY

Indisputably, QA is critical to modern medicine. The principals of evidence-based medicine and elimination of preventable harm are widely accepted. Although there is no longer disagreement (such as during Codman's time) about the importance of QA, there remains little consensus about the most effective means toward achieving these goals. It is important for the emergency physician to understand the current state of quality measurement in the ED, particularly the FPPE and OPPE processes as they affect individual providers. Future directions may include the development, validation, and implementation of more effective and efficient strategies for monitoring and reviewing quality of care, while simultaneously analyzing and characterizing contributing factors (provider, patient, system) to important care processes.

DISCLOSURE

W.E. Baker: Grant: 1R01HL127212 RACIAL AND ETHNIC HEALTH DISPARITIES DUE TO AMBULANCE DIVERSION. PI Hanchate, Amresh; Baker WE co-investigator). Funding from 1/15/2016 to 12/31/2019. Consultant: CRICO AMC/PSO. Provided emergency medicine subject matter expertise as part of risk assessment site visits of 2 separate EDs. Consultant: Cooney, Scully, and Dowling Attorneys. Provided emergency medicine expert witness services, medical malpractice case. Consultant: Boston HealthNet. Participated in physician panel for Boston HealthNet Plan Appeals Panel (credentials) hearing. J.J. Solano: #2018-01 Geriatric Head Trauma Short Term Outcome Project. PI Shih, RD; Alter, SM; Solano JJ co- investigators. Florida Medical Malpractice Joint Underwriting Association (FMMJUA) Alvin E. Smith Safety of Health Care Services Grant Program. Funding from 7/1/2019-6/30/2021.

REFERENCES

1. Codman EA. The classic: A study in hospital efficiency: as demonstrated by the case report of first five years of private hospital. Clin Orthop 2013;471(6):1778–83.
2. Codman EA. A study in hospital efficiency: as demonstrated by the case report of the first five years of a private hospital. Codman Hospital. Boston: Th Codman Co; 1918.
3. Levy R, Goldstein B, Trott A. Approach to quality assurance in an emergency department: A one-year review. Ann Emerg Med 1984;13(3):166–9.
4. Institute of Medicine (US), Committee on Quality of Health Care in America. In: Kohn LT, Corrigan JM, Donaldson MS, editors. To Err is human: building a safer health system. Washington, DC: National Academies Press (US); 2000. Available at: http://www.ncbi.nlm.nih.gov/books/NBK225182/. Accessed October 13, 2019.
5. FastStats. 2019. Available at: https://www.cdc.gov/nchs/fastats/emergency-department.htm. Accessed January 18, 2020.
6. Timely & Effective Care. Available at: https://www.medicare.gov/hospitalcompare/About/Timely-Effective-Care.html. Accessed January 18, 2020.
7. Institute of Medicine (US), Committee to Design a Strategy for Quality Review and Assurance in Medicare. In: Lohr KN, editor. Medicare: a strategy for quality assurance: VOLUME II sources and methods. Washington, DC: National Academies Press (US); 1990. Available at: http://www.ncbi.nlm.nih.gov/books/NBK235470/. Accessed January 18, 2020.
8. Institute of Medicine (US), Committee on Quality of Health Care in America. Crossing the quality Chasm: a new health system for the 21st century. Washington, DC: National Academies Press (US); 2001. Available at: http://www.ncbi.nlm.nih.gov/books/NBK222274/. Accessed October 20, 2019.
9. Six Domains of Health Care Quality. Available at: http://www.ahrq.gov/talkingquality/measures/six-domains.html. Accessed January 18, 2020.
10. Reason J. Human Error. Cambridge Core. https://doi.org/10.1017/CBO9781139062367.
11. 2011 report to Congress: national strategy for quality improvement in health care. Available at: https://www.ahrq.gov/workingforquality/reports/2011-annual-report.html. Accessed October 5, 2019.
12. Smith JM. EMTALA basics: what medical professionals need to know. Emergency Medical Treatment and Active Labor Act. J Natl Med Assoc 2002;94(6):426–9.
13. Terp S, Wang B, Raffetto B, et al. Individual physician penalties resulting from violation of emergency medical treatment and labor act: a review of office of the inspector general patient dumping settlements, 2002-2015. Acad Emerg Med 2017;24(4):442–6.
14. Keith KD, Bocka JJ, Kobernick MS, et al. Emergency department revisits. Ann Emerg Med 1989;18(9):964–8.
15. Flint LS, Hammett WH, Martens K. Quality assurance in the emergency department. Ann Emerg Med 1985;14(2):134–8.
16. Schwartz LR, Overton DT. Emergency department complaints: A one-year analysis. Ann Emerg Med 1987;16(8):857–61.
17. Klasco RS, Wolfe RE, Wong M, et al. Assessing the rates of error and adverse events in the ED. Am J Emerg Med 2015;33(12):1786–9.
18. Solano JJ, Dubosh NM, Anderson PD, et al. Hospital ward transfer to intensive care unit as a quality marker in emergency medicine. Am J Emerg Med 2017; 35(5):753–6.

19. Klasco RS, Wolfe RE, Lee T, et al. Can medical record reviewers reliably identify errors and adverse events in the ED? Am J Emerg Med 2016;34(6):1043–8.

20. Foley EM, Wolfe RE, Burstein JL, et al. Utility of procedural sedation as a marker for quality assurance in emergency medicine. J Emerg Med 2016;50(5):711–4.

21. Griffey RT, Schneider RM, Sharp BR, et al. Description and yield of current quality and safety review in selected US academic emergency departments. J Patient Saf 2017;1. https://doi.org/10.1097/PTS.0000000000000379.

22. Classen DC, Resar R, Griffin F, et al. "Global trigger tool" shows that adverse events in hospitals may be ten times greater than previously measured. Health Aff (Millwood) 2011;30(4):581–9.

23. Accreditation Council for Graduate Medical Education. ACGME Common Program Requirements (Residency). 2019. Available at: https://www.acgme.org/What-We-Do/Accreditation/Common-Program-Requirements. Accessed November 1, 2019.

24. Writing Committee Members, Antman EM, Anbe DT, et al. ACC/AHA Guidelines for the Management of Patients With ST-Elevation Myocardial Infarction—Executive Summary: A Report of the American College of Cardiology/American Heart Association Task Force on Practice Guidelines (Writing Committee to Revise the 1999 Guidelines for the Management of Patients With Acute Myocardial Infarction). Circulation 2004;110(5):588–636.

25. O'Gara PT, Kushner FG, Ascheim DD, et al. 2013 ACCF/AHA guideline for the management of ST-elevation myocardial infarction. J Am Coll Cardiol 2013; 61(4):e78–140.

26. Recommendations for Criteria for STEMI Systems of Care. Available at: http://www.heart.org/HEARTORG/HealthcareProfessional/Mission-Lifeline-Recommendations-for-Criteria-for-STEMI-Systems-of-Care_UCM_312070_Article.jsp#.XeSARr97mjR. Accessed December 1, 2019.

27. Walls RM, Resnick J. The joint commission on accreditation of healthcare organizations and center for medicare and medicaid services community-acquired pneumonia initiative: what went wrong? Ann Emerg Med 2005;46(5):409–11.

28. NQF: National Voluntary Consensus Standards for Emergency Care. Available at: http://www.qualityforum.org/Publications/2009/09/National_Voluntary_Consensus_Standards_for_Emergency_Care.aspx. Accessed October 5, 2019.

29. Venkatesh AK, Goodrich K. Emergency care and the national quality strategy: highlights from the centers for medicare & medicaid services. Ann Emerg Med 2015;65(4):396–9.

30. Schuur JD, Hsia RY, Burstin H, et al. Quality measurement in the emergency department: past and future. Health Aff (Millwood) 2013;32(12):2129–38.

31. Spivack SB, Laugesen MJ, Oberlander J. No permanent fix: MACRA, MIPS, and the politics of physician payment reform. J Health Polit Policy Law 2018;43(6): 1025–40.

32. CEDR. Available at: http://www.acep.org/cedr/. Accessed October 25, 2019.

33. Evolving emergency care with technology and data driven quality. Available at: http://www.acep.org/cedr/newsroom/2019/evolving-emergency-care-with-technology-and-data-driven-quality/. Accessed October 25, 2019.

34. E-QUAL Network FAQ. Available at: http://www.acep.org/administration/quality/equal/emergency-quality-network-e-qual/acep-e-qual-network-faq/. Accessed October 26, 2019.

35. Griffey RT, Pines JM, Farley HL, et al. Chief complaint–based performance measures: a new focus for acute care quality measurement. Ann Emerg Med 2015; 65(4):387–95.

36. Pregnancy Test for Female Abdominal Pain Patients (ACEP-24). Available at: http://www.acep.org/cedr/newsroom/2019/pregnancy-test-for-female-abdominal-pain-patients–acep-24/. Accessed October 26, 2019.

37. Raja AS, Walls RM, Schuur JD. Decreasing use of high-cost imaging: the danger of utilization-based performance measures. Ann Emerg Med 2010;56(6):597–9.

38. Coding Trends of Medicare Evaluation and Management Services (OEI-04-10-00180; 05/12). 39.

39. Care I of M (US) and NA of E (US) R on V& S-DH. Healthcare system complexities, impediments, and failures. Washington (US): National Academies Press; 2011. Available at: http://www.ncbi.nlm.nih.gov/books/NBK61963/. Accessed October 26, 2019.

40. Farley H, Enguidanos ER, Coletti CM, et al. Patient Satisfaction Surveys and Quality of Care: An Information Paper. Ann Emerg Med 2014;64(4):351–7.

41. Department of Health & Human Services Centers for Medicare & Medicaid Services. Conditions of Participation for Hospitals. Vol CFR §482. 2008. Available at: https://www.cms.gov/Regulations-and-Guidance/Guidance/Transmittals/downloads/R37SOMA.pdf. Accessed November 1, 2019.

42. Centers for Medicare and Medicaid Services. Quality, Safety & Oversight - Certification & Compliance. Hospitals. 2019. Available at: https://www.cms.gov/Medicare/Provider-Enrollment-and-Certification/CertificationandComplianc/Hospitals.html. Accessed November 1, 2019.

43. The Joint Commission. Facts about Hospital Accreditation. Available at: https://www.jointcommission.org/facts_about_hospital_accreditation/. Accessed November 1, 2019.

44. The Joint Commission. Medical Staff. In: The Joint commission comprehensive accreditation and certification manual, E-Dition. Oak Brook (IL): Joint Commission Resources; 2019. Available at: https://e-dition.jcrinc.com/MainContent.aspx. Accessed October 25, 2019.

45. Based on Core Competencies | American Board of Medical Specialties. Available at: https://www.abms.org/board-certification/a-trusted-credential/based-on-core-competencies/. Accessed November 1, 2019.

46. The Joint Commission. What is the intent of the requirement for Ongoing Professional Practice Evaluation? Standards FAQ Details. Available at: https://www.jointcommission.org/standards_information/jcfaqdetails.aspx. Accessed October 22, 2019.

47. The Joint Commission. Focused Professional Practice Evaluation (FPPE)- Four Required Components. Available at: https://www.jointcommission.org/standards_information/jcfaqdetails.aspx. Accessed October 7, 2019.

48. The Joint Commission. What is the duration of the monitoring? Focused Professional Practice Evaluation (FPPE) - Monitoring Timeline. Available at: https://www.jointcommission.org/standards_information/jcfaqdetails.aspx. Accessed October 26, 2019.

49. The Joint Commission. Ongoing Professional Practice Evaluation (OPPE) - Medical/Cognitive Specialties. Available at: https://www.jointcommission.org/standards_information/jcfaqdetails.aspx. Accessed November 1, 2019.

50. The Joint Commission. Ongoing Professional Practice Evaluation (OPPE) - Data Collection Guidelines and Frequency. Available at: https://www.jointcommission.org/mobile/standards_information/jcfaqdetails.aspx?StandardsFAQId=1879&StandardsFAQChapterId=25&ProgramId=0&ChapterId=0&IsFeatured=False&IsNew=False&Keyword=. Accessed October 26, 2019.

51. Kazandjian VA, Lawthers J, Cernak CM, et al. Relating outcomes to processes of care: the Maryland Hospital Association's Quality Indicator Project (QI Project). Jt Comm J Qual Improv 1993;19(11):530–8.

52. Griffin F, Resar R. IHI global trigger tool for measuring adverse events. 2nd edition. Cambridge (MA): Institute for Healthcare Improvement; 2009. Available at: www.IHI.org.

53. Boonyasai RT, Ijagbemi OM, Pham JC, et al. Improving the Emergency Department Discharge Process: Environmental Scan Report. Rockville (MD): Agency for Healthcare Research and Quality; :50. Available at: https://www.ahrq.gov/sites/default/files/wysiwyg/professionals/systems/hospital/edenvironmentalscan/edenvironmentalscan.pdf. Accessed November 17, 2019.

54. Rising KL, Victor TW, Hollander JE, et al. Patient returns to the emergency department: the time-to-return curve. Acad Emerg Med 2014;21(8):864–71.

55. Rising KL, Padrez KA, O'Brien M, et al. Return visits to the emergency department: the patient perspective. Ann Emerg Med 2015;65(4):377–86.e3.

56. Sabbatini AK, Kocher KE, Basu A, et al. In-hospital outcomes and costs among patients hospitalized during a return visit to the emergency department. JAMA 2016;315(7):663–71.

57. Cheng J, Shroff A, Khan N, et al. Emergency department return visits resulting in admission: do they reflect quality of care? Am J Med Qual 2016;31(6):541–51.

58. Aaronson E, Borczuk P, Benzer T, et al. 72h returns: A trigger tool for diagnostic error. Am J Emerg Med 2018;36(3):359–61.

59. Walker LE, Phelan MP, Bitner M, et al. Ongoing and focused provider performance evaluations in emergency medicine: current practices and modified delphi to guide future practice. Am J Med Qual 2019. https://doi.org/10.1177/1062860619874113. 1062860619874113.

60. Flowerdew L, Brown R, Vincent C, et al. Identifying nontechnical skills associated with safety in the emergency department: a scoping review of the literature. Ann Emerg Med 2012;59(5):386–94.

61. Daouk-Öyry L, Mufarrij A, Khalil M, et al. Nurse-led competency model for emergency physicians: a qualitative study. Ann Emerg Med 2017;70(3):357–62.e5.

62. Flowerdew L, Brown R, Vincent C, et al. Development and validation of a tool to assess emergency physicians' nontechnical skills. Ann Emerg Med 2012;59(5):376–85.e4.

63. Institute of Medicine (US) Committee to Design a Strategy for Quality Review and Assurance in Medicare. In: Aspden P, Corrigan JM, Wolcott J, et al, editors. Patient safety: achieving a new standard for care. Washington, DC: The National Academies Press; 2004. Available at: https://www.nap.edu/catalog/10863/patient-safety-achieving-a-new-standard-for-care. Accessed November 24, 2019.

64. Sherman H, Castro G, Fletcher M, et al. Towards an International Classification for Patient Safety: the conceptual framework. Int J Qual Health Care 2009;21(1):2–8.

65. Chang A, Schyve PM, Croteau RJ, et al. The JCAHO patient safety event taxonomy: a standardized terminology and classification schema for near misses and adverse events. Int J Qual Health Care 2005;17(2):95–105.

66. The Joint Commission. Sentinel event policy and procedures 2019. Available at: https://www.jointcommission.org/sentinel_event_policy_and_procedures/. Accessed November 24, 2019.

67. Hartwig SC, Denger SD, Schneider PJ. Severity-indexed, incident report-based medication error-reporting program. Am J Hosp Pharm 1991;48(12):2611–6.

68. National coordinating Council for medication error reporting and Prevention (NCC MERP). NCC MERP taxonomy of medication errors. National Coordinating Council for Medication Error Reporting and Prevention; 1998. Available at: https://www.nccmerp.org/taxonomy-medication-errors-now-available. Accessed November 21, 2019.

69. Agency for Healthcare Research and Quality. Extent of harm. U.S. Department of Health & Human Services; 2013. Available at: https://ushik.ahrq.gov/ViewItemDetails?&system=ps&itemKey=169080000. Accessed November 24, 2019.

70. Hoppes M, Mitchell J. Serious safety events: a focus on harm Classification: deviation in care as link getting to ZeroTM white paper Series — edition No. 2. Chicago: American Society for Healthcare Risk Management; 2014.

71. Taylor-Adams S, Vincent C. Systems analysis of clinical incidents: the London protocol. Clin Risk 2004;10(6):211–20.

72. Dekker S. The field guide to understanding "human error." 3 edition. Farnham, Surrey, England. Burlington (VT): Routledge; 2014.

73. Dahn CM, Manasco AT, Breaud AH, et al. A critical analysis of unplanned ICU transfer within 48 hours from ED admission as a quality measure. Am J Emerg Med 2016;34(8):1505–10.

74. Griffey RT, Schneider RM, Todorov AA. The emergency department trigger tool: a novel approach to screening for quality and safety events. Ann Emerg Med 2019. https://doi.org/10.1016/j.annemergmed.2019.07.032.

Information Management in the Emergency Department

Evan L. Leventhal, MD, PhD[a],*, Kraftin E. Schreyer, MD[b]

KEYWORDS

- Electronic medical records • Emergency department information systems
- Communication • Informatics • Operations

KEY POINTS

- Communication in the emergency department (ED) takes many forms, and clear communication is critical to successful patient care.
- Interruptive alerts should be used sparingly and only for the most severe or high-risk alarms.
- Systems must be developed to detect and remove or correct low-yield alerts in order to minimize alert fatigue.
- Additional research is needed on ED information systems and ED-specific communication.
- The future of information management should largely focus on minimizing interruptions, improving provider wellness, and reducing provider burnout.

INTRODUCTION

The emergency department (ED) is a unique health care environment. It is complex, unpredictable, resource limited, and constantly in flux.[1] The amount of information that must be managed to adequately and safely care for patients in the ED can be overwhelming. This information must not only be identified, documented, interpreted, and retrieved but often it needs to be communicated and acted on immediately. The communication burden on ED providers is unbounded and fraught with interruptions and distractions that potentially introduce error and lead to mismanagement of information.

The percentage of hospitals with an electronic medical record (EMR) has increased over the past decade. As of 2017, 96% of acute care hospitals possessed certified

The authors contributed equally to this work and are listed alphabetically.
[a] Department of Emergency Medicine, Beth Israel Deaconess Medical Center, Harvard Medical School, 1 Deaconess Road, Boston, MA 02215, USA; [b] Department of Emergency Medicine, Temple University Hospital, Lewis Katz School of Medicine at Temple University, Philadelphia, PA 19140, USA
* Corresponding author.
E-mail address: eleventh@bidmc.harvard.edu

https://doi.org/10.1016/j.emc.2020.03.004
emed.theclinics.com

EMRs.[2] This article refers to the interface of the EMR used by ED providers as ED information systems (EDISs). Although many health care systems use a dedicated interface for the EDIS, others use the same interface and layout as the inpatient providers.

EDISs are not perfect systems. They help manage the vast amount of information in an ED but have been shown to both benefit and harm ED patient care.[3] EDIS workflows are often time intensive and detract from other tasks, including provider-patient interactions.[4] In addition to impeding throughput, EDISs have the potential to introduce new forms of error into the system, and the burden of electronic documentation can lead to provider burnout.[4,5]

COMMUNICATION IN THE EMERGENCY DEPARTMENT

Communication is paramount to the delivery of safe, high-quality, effective, and efficient care in any ED.[1,6,7] Successful communication is a combination of active and passive communication techniques, and takes many forms.[6] Each form of communication involves both the transfer of information but also behaviors accompanying that transfer.[6]

The communication load on emergency providers has been shown to be substantial. It has been estimated that communication, in all its forms, occupies about 80% of clinicians' time.[8] Coiera and colleagues[9] found that a third of communication events were interruptions, and, 10% of the time, communications involved more than 1 simultaneous conversation. This volume of communication can be problematic in many ways. The sheer volume of communication can overwhelm short-term memory, causing more relevant pieces of information to be forgotten. Untimely or irrelevant data are distracting and interrupt workflow, including complex decision making and task performance.[8] Observational studies have shown clinicians in the ED are interrupted as frequently as every 6 to 9 minutes.[10] The enormous amount of communication that takes place in a complex, high-risk environment such as an ED has the potential to directly contribute to medical errors, adverse events, and patient harm.[6]

Modes of Communication

Fairbanks and colleagues[9] identified several modes of communication in the ED setting (**Box 1**). Face-to-face communication has been shown to be the most common form of communication in an ED, estimated to be from 82% to 90% of all communication.[8,9,11]

The advent of secure texting systems has substantially expanded transmission of patient information for consultation, admission, or other transitions of care. As a result, mobile phones have increasingly supplanted the more traditional communication modality of paging, although personal and overhead pagers are still used in many EDs. Overhead announcements are still used throughout many EDs to communicate a multitude of information, including patient arrivals, notification of needed tests (ie, electrocardiograms or radiographs), and to alert ancillary personnel of the need for their service.[7]

With the advent of the EMR, computers are growing as a fundamental communication tool, but one with new benefits and potential pitfalls. EMRs allow for a wide range of communication modalities, including messaging platforms, push notifications, and automated and asynchronous messages such as best-practice alerts (BPAs).

EMERGENCY DEPARTMENT INFORMATION SYSTEMS

As part of the Centers for Medicare and Medicaid Services meaningful use criteria, hospitals in the United States are now required to use certified EMRs and EDIS.[12]

Box 1
Common forms of communication within the emergency department

- Face to face
- Telephone
- Chart writing and reading
- Order writing and reading
- Whiteboards
- Test and laboratory results
- Item drop-off (eg, Sticky note)
- Vitals (on a monitor)
- Computer
- Other

Data from Coiera EW, Jayasuriya RA, Hardy J, et al. Communication loads on clinical staff in the emergency department. Med J Aust. 2002;176(9):415-418.

Most EMRs are chosen by health system administrators. EMRs have increased the frequency of task switching that providers perform,[13] with physicians clicking the mouse almost 4000 times in a single shift.[14] This increase in workload and the frequency of interruptions has increased the risk of new types of medical errors, which both threaten patient safety and also contribute to provider burnout.[15] Physicians now spend 25% to 65% of their time during a shift documenting.[16,17]

Not surprisingly, providers often find EMRs difficult to use.[13] EMRs often have busy, confusing displays that attempt to cram large amounts of information in a small space. Data organization within the EMR often does not match clinical workflow, resulting in information remaining undiscovered.[18] Furthermore, different ED team members may have different screen layouts or access to different areas of the chart, increasing the potential for miscommunication.[19]

To address some of those issues, some health systems have standardized their EMR layout for all members of the health care team. Other systems give the option of direct communication between providers within the EMR.[19] Additional recommended improvements include reducing variability within the EMR, standardizing provider interaction with the EMR, formal usability assessments, and adverse events reporting systems.[14]

In spite of the problems that they have been shown to cause for providers, EDISs have proved to be valuable tools for accumulating and storing data specific to both patients and the ED. These data can be used in real time by clinical staff or administrative leaders to identify and troubleshoot problems in flow (eg, radiology or laboratory delays, overcrowding, or an influx of patients), and can also be used retrospectively for research and quality-improvement purposes.[3]

INPUT
Prehospital

Emergency medical service (EMS) arrivals, especially those for patients with time-sensitive clinical conditions, can be preceded by a prehospital notification that readies providers.[20] EMS providers are a source of valuable information, but information is frequently lost during this handoff, especially for lower-acuity patients. In particular, the lack of a standardized handoff process from EMS to nursing can lead to failures in communicating patient needs and expectations.[21] These omissions can subsequently result in impaired ED flow, repetitive testing, or excessive work-ups. Although, in many EDs, EMS trip sheets are scanned into the EDIS, there is often a delay between the entry of these data and the patient's arrival, making them an unreliable source of information.[22]

Outpatient Referrals

An estimated 12% to 59% of patients have made contact with their outpatient providers before an ED visit or are referred to the ED.[23–26] Referrals from the outpatient team to the ED can come in many forms, including verbal handoffs to either triage nurses or ED providers, paperwork sent with the patient, a note within the hospital EMR or EDIS, or an electronic message sent directly to the ED. An electronic referral that is automatically associated with the patient in the EDIS intuitively seems like the best option for many ED providers; however, there is limited research in this area. Many hospitals also send notifications to primary care providers when patients are registered within the ED.[27]

Triage

Although standardized triage scores and criteria are common in the ED, there is considerable variability in the information documented in different hospitals' EDISs during the triage process. Universally collected information includes the patients' chief complaints and vital signs. Other information, including past medical and surgical history, social history, medication reconciliation, allergies, and screenings for abuse or public health measures, can be collected during the initial triage phase but can also be collected later in a patient's ED stay.[28] Some of the heterogeneity of information gathered in triage is caused by the triage process being presented differently in different EDISs. However, regulatory requirements for gathering information can place an undue burden on triage, resulting in poor signal/noise ratio and information being either hidden or overlooked.[29]

Increased morbidity and mortality can result from triage errors, including overtriage and undertriage.[30] In addition, care trajectories can often be altered if the information in triage is incorrect or overlooked.[29] Further complicating information management in triage is the simple fact that patients may tell triage nurses something about their presentation that they do not repeat later in their ED stays. If those particular details are not incorporated into the initial triage assessment, they may never be reclaimed. Both the variability of the information gathered in triage and the location of that information within the EDIS make managing triage information challenging for ED providers.

Patient identification

The handling of unidentified patients in the ED is a frequent occurrence. Numerous schemes have been developed for how to represent these individuals.[23,31,32] This requirement is especially important when there are large numbers of unknown patients in the department (eg, mass casualty incidents). Recommended strategies include visually distinct representation with names that are unique and easy for providers to remember.[32]

Transgender patients deserve special attention. As an already marginalized group, the most basic single-step registration system, containing only a single binary field to represent gender, can cause problems for both patients and providers.[24] Although 2-step processes identifying a patient's gender identity and their birth-assigned sex improve on this process,[25] newer techniques have been suggested to collect a patient's gender identity (ie, how a patient wishes to be addressed), the birth sex, and the legal sex.[26] Whatever system is used, it is important that providers be able to easily identify transgender patients in order to provide the best care possible.

Notification of New Patients

Notification of new patient arrivals to the ED and of their subsequent placement in treatment spaces can happen through verbal and nonverbal means. Nonverbal communication typically takes the form of a change in the EDIS, such as a color change that reflects a patient's status or the appearance of the patient's name on a track board or map. Verbal communication could be face to face, if the charge nurse or triage nurse directly notifies a bedside nurse or provider of a new patient being bedded in their treatment area, or it could take the form of overhead pages or announcements.[7]

THROUGHPUT
Emergency Department Information System Chart Matching

Before electronic records, patients were often physically accompanied by their paper charts. In the current era of electronic records, it is common to have multiple patient charts open at once, and often patient names are not fully displayed between charts.[27] A simple misclick can lead a provider to the wrong patient's chart and, in turn, can lead to documentation and ordering errors.

Matching the correct chart is especially important in computerized physician order entry (CPOE) systems, where there is potential for harm by ordering inappropriate tests or interventions on the wrong patient. It has been suggested that the prominent display of the patient's room[12] as well as patient photographs[16] have the potential to prevent wrong-patient orders.

Emergency Department Information System Chart Review

It has been shown that providers spend about 12% of their time reviewing results and old records.[17] One of the manifest benefits of EDISs is that they have made old records more accessible for review and more comprehensive. Information can now be shared between hospitals and health systems, through improved interoperability and health information exchanges, although there remains a substantial disparity.[14,19] However, the amount of information now available can make finding relevant information more challenging and time consuming.

Computerized Physician Order Entry Systems

Development of CPOE was one of the earliest uses of EMRs and is well adopted. Its use has been shown to affect the communication pattern between providers and nurses.[13] CPOE has been shown to reduce the rate of medication errors,[33] and with reported high user satisfaction.[34]

Integrated allergy alerts and drug-drug interaction alerts are important features of CPOE, which have been shown to reduce adverse medication reactions in the ED.[33] As shown by providers overriding up to 90% of these alerts, most are clinically insignificant.[15] Having such a high false-positive rate of alerts creates a classic example of alert fatigue, where users become accustomed to ignoring these alerts and are more likely to overlook those with clinical significance that could negatively affect patient care.[35] It has thus been recommended that many of these interaction alerts should be noninterruptive.[36]

Order sets have been proposed as a method of both making it easier for providers to quickly place orders on their patients and standardizing care between providers, but there are variable rates of adherence with order sets.[13,37,38] ED-specific order sets and dashboards have been created to match key pieces of information with patient care flow.[13,33]

Best-Practice Alerts

BPAs are alerts within the EDIS to prompt intervention or inform the user. BPAs are clinical support tools designed to help improve safety, but they can also be used to reduce cost by reducing duplicate testing,[39,40] help remind providers to start antibiotics early in sepsis,[41] and decrease opioid prescribing.[42]

However, BPAs are often seen as a panacea for improving compliance metrics and other problems, leading to their overuse. This overuse has led to a marked increase in the number of alerts providers are faced with on a given shift, which in turn increases the burden of communication interruptions and changes in task they face. As the number of BPA alerts increases, providers become less likely to respond and more likely to ignore them, which is another example of alert fatigue. The rarer an event, the less useful BPAs become, which merits evaluation of other solutions and interventions.[39,43]

There have been various attempts to automatically detect when BPAs are incorrectly configured or are less useful. Aaron and colleagues[40] noted that users often responded with "cranky" free-text comments when overriding misconfigured alerts, and suggested that an automated detection system could be created to search for such cranky words.

Results

New results

Providers need to be made aware of new results in a timely manner. Most importantly, they need to be aware that all of the expected results have returned and the work-up is complete. Some systems have mechanisms by which the system can indicate that a patient has new results; however, in many implementations, this indicator can be reset the first time anyone reviews the results. These systems sometimes only indicate new results but do not indicate that all results are finalized. Other systems can indicate when all results are returned but can be confused by tests not anticipated to result during an ED visit (eg, cultures). Active notification of key results affecting disposition have been shown to decrease length of stay and improve patient flow.[41,44]

Interpreting results

Even though abnormal results are often displayed bolded or underlined, they can still be difficult to find and accidently overlooked.[45–49] Many EDISs list results in text or tabular format, rather than graphically. This format then requires providers to scroll through long lists of mostly normal results to identify and act on the abnormal results.[33] Failure to recognize these abnormal tests can negatively affect patient care.[48,49]

Critical results

Laboratory results are typically classified as within the normal, abnormal, or critical ranges. Critical results typically require confirmation that the information has been passed on.[50] Although most systems require verbal acknowledgment, critical results could alternatively be acknowledged through the EDIS. Only if the provider has failed to acknowledge the result in a certain time period would a follow-up verbal communication then be required. It has been proposed that critical results be further subdivided based on the timeliness of the clinical decision required.[51]

Patient portals

The increasing presence of patient-facing portals allows patients in the ED to view their records, including laboratory results and imaging data, on smartphones in real time. In many cases, patients are aware of their own results before the providing team, making for awkward interactions that providers should be prepared to address.[50]

Future work

In the future, it may be possible for the EMR to apply knowledge of the patient's condition to help determine what distinguishes a normal from an abnormal or critical result. For example, at a basic level, the normal range for a complete blood cell count could be appropriately adjusted for a patient in her third trimester. A more advanced system might recognize that a markedly increased lactate level in a patient presenting after a seizure is probably expected, and therefore should be flagged as merely abnormal as opposed to being communicated as a critical result.

OUTPUT
Admissions and Inpatient Handoff

Information management is particularly important during transitions of care. Handoffs between the ED and inpatient teams are a major source of medical error[52] and are complicated by the lack of a universal handoff process.[53] Transmission of inaccurate information was most commonly related to the physical examination, followed by the results of ancillary tests, the history of present illness, and the patients' clinical course while in the ED.[52]

Electronic asynchronous transitions of care have been used as an alternative to the traditional verbal handoff.[54] These models, which still allow for additional verbal communication when needed, are standardized and can help to minimize interruptions.[55] However, technology has also complicated ED-to-inpatient handoffs. Fragmented CPOE systems between the ED and inpatient units can make it difficult for inpatient providers to locate pending orders, resulting in duplication of work. When the EMR does not clearly delineate the current care team after a handoff, critical results can be communicated to the incorrect team.[52]

Discharge Communication

Clear discharge instructions are necessary to communicate to patients their diagnosis, treatment, follow-up plan, as well as return instructions.[56] It is recommended that these instructions be given both verbally as well as in written form. Multiple studies have shown that there are significant deficiencies in patient comprehension of their discharge instructions despite these efforts.[56–59] There are additional barriers for patients who speak different languages, as well as those with poor reading comprehension skills.[57,58,60] The use of interpreters to deliver verbal discharge instructions has been shown to be somewhat effective, although the amount of time spent with the patient is also important.[57]

Elderly patients being discharged back to a skilled nursing facility represent a particularly vulnerable population, especially when being discharged with a change in status, need for follow-up, or with new care instructions (eg, change in medication, new weight-bearing status, or new wound care instructions).[61]

In addition to individualized discharge instructions, it is important to have standardized instructions available in multiple languages.[57,62] The provider should be able to select the appropriate discharge instructions in the EMR, and the correct version should be automatically printed in the patient's preferred language.

SUMMARY AND RECOMMENDATIONS

Information management in the ED is complex and creates a large burden on providers, which hinders patient care. The future of information management should largely focus on minimizing interruptions, optimizing patient safety, and improving provider wellness. Based on our comprehensive review, we put forth the following recommendations:

1. A dedicated EDIS from the main EMR optimized for ED workflow
2. Standardization within the EDIS for the entire care team
3. Standardized and structured data collection at triage
4. Reservation of modal or interruptive alerts for only the most severe or high-risk alarms
5. Elimination of low-yield BPAs and alerts, and development of alternative solutions for intervening on rare events
6. Order sets and orders specific to ED care
7. Event-based notification for key positive and negative results that affect disposition or destination
8. A streamlined handoff process for admissions
9. Standardized discharge instructions
10. Further research dedicated to EDIS-specific and ED-specific communication

CONFLICTS OF INTEREST

The authors report no conflict of interest.

REFERENCES

1. Croskerry P, Sinclair D. Emergency medicine: A practice prone to error? CJEM 2001;3(4):271–6.
2. The United States Department of Health and Human Services (HHS), Office of the National Coordinator for Health Information Technology (ONC). 2018 Report to Congress - Annual Update on the Adoption of a Nationwide System for the Electronic Use and Exchange of Health Information. [internet]. https://www.healthit.gov/sites/default/files/page/2018-12/2018-HITECH-report-to-congress.pdf.
3. Taylor TB. Information management in the emergency department. Emerg Med Clin North Am 2004;22(1):241–57.
4. Kroth PJ, Morioka-Douglas N, Veres S, et al. The electronic elephant in the room: Physicians and the electronic health record. JAMIA Open 2018;1(1):49–56.
5. Downing NL, Bates DW, Longhurst CA. Physician burnout in the electronic health record era: are we ignoring the real cause? Ann Intern Med 2018;169(1):50.
6. Eisenberg EM, Murphy AG, Sutcliffe K, et al. Communication in Emergency Medicine: Implications for Patient Safety This study was funded by a generous grant from the National Patient Safety Foundation. Commun Monogr 2005;72(4):390–413.
7. Eng MS-B, Fierro K, Abdouche S, et al. Perceived vs. actual distractions in the emergency department. Am J Emerg Med 2019. https://doi.org/10.1016/j.ajem.2019.01.005.
8. Vincent CA, Wears RL. Communication in the emergency department: separating the signal from the noise. Med J Aust 2002;176(9):409–10.
9. Coiera EW, Jayasuriya RA, Hardy J, et al. Communication loads on clinical staff in the emergency department. Med J Aust 2002;176(9):415–8.
10. Kahn CA. Commentary: death by distraction. Ann Emerg Med 2016;68(2):234–5.

11. Fairbanks RJ, Bisantz AM, Sunm M. Emergency department communication links and patterns. Ann Emerg Med 2007;50(4):396–406.

12. Yamamoto LG. Reducing emergency department charting and ordering errors with a room number watermark on the electronic medical record display. Hawaii J Med Public Health 2014;73(10):322–8.

13. Asaro PV, Boxerman SB. Effects of computerized provider order entry and nursing documentation on workflow. Acad Emerg Med 2008;15(10):908–15.

14. Winden T, Boland L, Frey N, et al. Care everywhere, a point-to-point HIE tool. Appl Clin Inform 2014;05(02):388–401.

15. van der Sijs H, Aarts J, Vulto A, et al. Overriding of drug safety alerts in computerized physician order entry. J Am Med Inform Assoc 2006;13(2):138–47.

16. Hyman D, Laire M, Redmond D, et al. The use of patient pictures and verification screens to reduce computerized provider order entry errors. Pediatrics 2012; 130(1):e211–9.

17. Hill RG, Sears LM, Melanson SW. 4000 Clicks: a productivity analysis of electronic medical records in a community hospital ED. Am J Emerg Med 2013;31(11): 1591–4.

18. Bowman S. Impact of electronic health record systems on information integrity: quality and safety implications. Perspect Health Inf Manag 2013;10:1c.

19. Everson J, Kocher KE, Adler-Milstein J. Health information exchange associated with improved emergency department care through faster accessing of patient information from outside organizations. J Am Med Inform Assoc 2017;24(e1): e103–10.

20. Patel Mehul D, Rose Kathryn M, O'Brien Emily C, et al. Prehospital notification by emergency medical services reduces delays in stroke evaluation. Stroke 2011; 42(8):2263–8.

21. Reay G, Norris JM, Alix Hayden K, et al. Transition in care from paramedics to emergency department nurses: a systematic review protocol. Syst Rev 2017;6. https://doi.org/10.1186/s13643-017-0651-z.

22. Meisel ZF, Shea JA, Peacock NJ, et al. Optimizing the patient handoff between emergency medical services and the emergency department. Ann Emerg Med 2015;65(3):310–7.e1.

23. Robinson G, Fortune JB, Wachtel TL, et al. A system of alias assignment for unidentified patients requiring emergency hospital admission. J Trauma 1985;25(4): 333–6.

24. Safer JD, Coleman E, Feldman J, et al. Barriers to health care for transgender individuals. Curr Opin Endocrinol Diabetes Obes 2016;23(2):168–71.

25. Deutsch MB, Green J, Keatley J, et al. Electronic medical records and the transgender patient: recommendations from the World Professional Association for Transgender Health EMR Working Group. J Am Med Inform Assoc 2013;20(4): 700–3.

26. Deutsch MB, Buchholz D. Electronic health records and transgender patients— practical recommendations for the collection of gender identity data. J Gen Intern Med 2015;30(6):843–7.

27. Adelman JS, Berger MA, Rai A, et al. A national survey assessing the number of records allowed open in electronic health records at hospitals and ambulatory sites. J Am Med Inform Assoc 2017;24(5):992–5.

28. Castner J. Emergency Department triage: what data are nurses collecting? J Emerg Nurs 2011;37:417–22.

29. Upadhyay DK, Sittig DF, Singh H. Ebola US Patient Zero: lessons on misdiagnosis and effective use of electronic health records. Diagnosis (Berl) 2014;1(4):283–7.

30. Hinson JS, Martinez DA, Schmitz PSK, et al. Accuracy of emergency department triage using the Emergency Severity Index and independent predictors of under-triage and over-triage in Brazil: a retrospective cohort analysis. Int J Emerg Med 2018;11. https://doi.org/10.1186/s12245-017-0161-8.

31. Brooks AJ, Macnab C, Boffard K. AKA unknown male Foxtrot 23/4: alias assignment for unidentified emergency room patients. J Accid Emerg Med 1999;16(3): 171–3.

32. Landman A, Teich JM, Pruitt P, et al. The Boston Marathon bombings mass casualty incident: one emergency department's information systems challenges and opportunities. Ann Emerg Med 2015;66(1):51–9.

33. Bates DW, Teich JM, Lee J, et al. The impact of computerized physician order entry on medication error prevention. J Am Med Inform Assoc 1999;6(4):313–21.

34. Lee F, Teich JM, Spurr CD, et al. Implementation of physician order entry: user satisfaction and self-reported usage patterns. J Am Med Inform Assoc 1996; 3(1):42–55.

35. Embi PJ, Leonard AC. Evaluating alert fatigue over time to EHR-based clinical trial alerts: findings from a randomized controlled study. J Am Med Inform Assoc 2012;19(e1):e145–8.

36. Phansalkar S, van der Sijs H, Tucker AD, et al. Drug—drug interactions that should be non-interruptive in order to reduce alert fatigue in electronic health records. J Am Med Inform Assoc 2013;20(3):489–93.

37. Reingold S, Kulstad E. Impact of human factor design on the use of order sets in the treatment of congestive heart failure. Acad Emerg Med 2007;14(11): 1097–105.

38. Li RC, Wang JK, Sharp C, et al. When order sets do not align with clinician workflow: assessing practice patterns in the electronic health record. BMJ Qual Saf 2019. https://doi.org/10.1136/bmjqs-2018-008968. bmjqs-2018-008968.

39. Ancker JS, Edwards A, Nosal S, et al. Effects of workload, work complexity, and repeated alerts on alert fatigue in a clinical decision support system. BMC Med Inform Decis Mak 2017;17(1):36.

40. Aaron S, McEvoy DS, Ray S, et al. Cranky comments: detecting clinical decision support malfunctions through free-text override reasons. J Am Med Inform Assoc 2018;26(1):37–43.

41. Verma A, Wang AS, Feldman MJ, et al. Push-alert notification of troponin results to physician smartphones reduces the time to discharge emergency department patients: a randomized controlled trial. Ann Emerg Med 2017;70(3):348–56.

42. Malte CA, Berger D, Saxon AJ, et al. Electronic medical record alert associated with reduced opioid and benzodiazepine coprescribing in high-risk veteran patients. Med Care 2018;56(2):171–8.

43. Chen H, Butler E, Guo Y, et al. Facilitation or hindrance: physicians' perception on best practice alerts (BPA) usage in an electronic health record system. Health Commun 2019;34(9):942–8.

44. Salmasian H, Landman AB, Morris C. An electronic notification system for improving patient flow in the emergency department. AMIA Jt Summits Transl Sci Proc 2019;2019:242–7.

45. Duncan BJ, Zheng L, Furniss SK, et al. In search of vital signs: a comparative study of EHR documentation. AMIA Annu Symp Proc 2018;2018:1233–42.

46. Farley HL, Baumlin KM, Hamedani AG, et al. Quality and safety implications of emergency department information systems. Ann Emerg Med 2013;62(4): 399–407.

47. El-Kareh R, Pazo V, Wright A, et al. Losing weights: Failure to recognize and act on weight loss documented in an electronic health record. J Innov Health Inform 2015;22(3):316–22.
48. Callen J, Giardina TD, Singh H, et al. Emergency physicians' views of direct notification of laboratory and radiology results to patients using the internet: a multisite survey. J Med Internet Res 2015;17(3). https://doi.org/10.2196/jmir.3721.
49. Kachalia A, Gandhi TK, Puopolo AL, et al. Missed and delayed diagnoses in the emergency department: a study of closed malpractice claims from 4 liability insurers. Ann Emerg Med 2007;49(2):196–205.
50. Dighe AS, Rao A, Coakley AB, et al. Analysis of laboratory critical value reporting at a large academic medical center. Am J Clin Pathol 2006;125(5):758–64.
51. Hanna D, Griswold P, Leape LL, et al. Communicating critical test results: safe practice recommendations. Jt Comm J Qual Patient Saf 2005;31(2):68–80.
52. Horwitz LI, Meredith T, Schuur JD, et al. Dropping the baton: a qualitative analysis of failures during the transition from emergency department to inpatient care. Ann Emerg Med 2009;53(6):701–10.e4.
53. McFetridge B, Gillespie M, Goode D, et al. An exploration of the handover process of critically ill patients between nursing staff from the emergency department and the intensive care unit. Nurs Crit Care 2007;12(6):261–9.
54. Sanchez LD, Chiu DT, Nathanson L, et al. A model for electronic handoff between the emergency department and inpatient units. J Emerg Med 2017;53(1):142–50.
55. Ortiz-Figueroa F. Efficiency of electronic signout for ED-to-inpatient admission at a non-teaching hospital commentary. Intern Emerg Med 2018;13(7):1103–4.
56. Hoek AE, Anker SCP, van Beeck EF, et al. Patient discharge instructions in the emergency department and their effects on comprehension and recall of discharge instructions: a systematic review and meta-analysis. Ann Emerg Med 2019. https://doi.org/10.1016/j.annemergmed.2019.06.008.
57. Samuels-Kalow ME, Stack AM, Porter SC. Effective discharge communication in the emergency department. Ann Emerg Med 2012;60(2):152–9.
58. Glick AF, Farkas JS, Nicholson J, et al. Parental management of discharge instructions: a systematic review. Pediatrics 2017;140(2). https://doi.org/10.1542/peds.2016-4165.
59. Hess DR, Tokarczyk A, O'Malley M, et al. The value of adding a verbal report to written handoffs on early readmission following prolonged respiratory failure. Chest 2010;138(6):1475–9.
60. Karliner LS, Auerbach A, Nápoles A, et al. Language barriers and understanding of hospital discharge instructions. Med Care 2012;50(4):283–9.
61. King BJ, Gilmore-Bykovskyi AL, Roiland RA, et al. The consequences of poor communication during transitions from hospital to skilled nursing facility: a qualitative study. J Am Geriatr Soc 2013;61(7):1095–102.
62. Vukmir RB, Kremen R, Dehart DA, et al. Compliance with emergency department patient referral. Am J Emerg Med 1992;10(5):413–7.

Best Practices in Patient Safety and Communication

Dana Im, MD, MPP, MPhil[a],*, Emily Aaronson, MD, MPH[b]

KEYWORDS

- Patient safety • Emergency medicine • Communication • Teamwork

KEY POINTS

- Emergency departments are high-risk practice environments, with a high rate of preventable adverse events.
- Teamwork and communication are key drivers for safe care.
- Best practices for improving patient safety can be framed around (1) cultivating safety culture, (2) implementing processes to improve patient safety, and (3) creating systems-based approaches to patient safety.

INTRODUCTION

The Institute of Medicine's (IOM) 1999 report, *To Err is Human: Building a Safer Health System*, increased awareness of medical errors in the United States, highlighting patient safety concerns as a serious public health issue. Based on 2 large retrospective studies, the report estimated 44,000 to 98,000 deaths per year in the United States occurring as a result of medical errors.[1]

- The Harvard Medical Practice Study, a population-based estimate of adverse events in hospitals in New York, found that adverse events occurred in 3.7% of hospitalizations, of which 27.6% were from negligence and 13.6% were fatal events.[2]
- The Colorado–Utah Study showed that adverse events occurred in 2.9% of nonpsychiatric hospitalizations. Of all the adverse events, 27.4% in Utah and 32.5% in Colorado were considered negligent adverse events. Approximately 9% of all negligent adverse events were fatal.[3]

Both studies reported that the emergency department (ED) had the highest proportion of adverse events caused by negligence.[2–4] Evidence suggests that between 6.0% and 8.5% of the patients who receive care in the ED experience an adverse

[a] Department of Emergency Medicine, Brigham and Women's Hospital, 75 Francis Street, NH-2, Boston, MA 02115, USA; [b] Massachusetts General Hospital, 55 Fruit Street, Bulfinch 290, Boston, MA 02114, USA
* Corresponding author.
E-mail address: dim@partners.org

Emerg Med Clin N Am 38 (2020) 693–703
https://doi.org/10.1016/j.emc.2020.04.007
0733-8627/20/Published by Elsevier Inc.
emed.theclinics.com

event.[5,6] The majority of adverse events occurring in the ED are believed to be preventable.[3,7] Caring for patients in the emergency setting is considered particularly prone to adverse events because of factors inherent to the task of delivering emergency care (summarized in **Table 1**). At all risk levels – provider, patient, and environmental levels—medical errors predominantly arise from system and process issues, rather than individual human failures.

Although the IOM report focused the attention of the US public on the magnitude of medical errors, it also created a window of opportunity to improve patient safety. Patient safety, defined as "the prevention of errors and adverse effects to patients associated with health care," has become a priority issue for health care professionals, policymakers, accrediting agencies, and patients and families.[20] Although medical errors can happen despite people's best efforts, health care professionals must be proactive about improving patient safety in the emergency care system.

FRAMEWORK FOR IMPROVING PATIENT SAFETY AND COMMUNICATION IN THE EMERGENCY DEPARTMENT

In this section, we propose a conceptual framework that describes the best practices for improving patient safety in the ED. The framework consists of 3 major domains: (1) cultivating safety culture, (2) implementing processes to improve patient safety, and (3) creating systems-based approaches to patient safety (**Fig. 1**).

Cultivating Safety Culture

Establishing safety culture is the basic foundation of achieving sustainable improvements in patient safety. Safety culture has been defined as "the product of individual and group beliefs, values, attitudes, perceptions, competencies, and patterns of behavior that determine the organization's commitment to quality and patient safety,"[21] with the goal of making patient safety everyone's highest priority.[22] The goal of a culture of safety is to make the ED a high reliability organization, an organization that can operate complex systems in a high-risk environment while maintaining very low rates of harm and errors.[23,24] High reliability organizations can strive for improvement in patient safety through a collective desire to achieve perfect while fostering mutual understanding among its members that a mishap can occur at any time, and that no one individual or organization is at fault when medical errors do occur.[23]

Table 1	
Levels of risk factors associated with adverse events in the ED	
Levels of Risks	**Risk Factors**
Provider level	Disrupted sleep cycle[8–12]
	Cognitive overload[13]
	Communication breakdowns with transfer of care/signout[11,14]
Patient level	Patient acuity and complexity, under unpredictable conditions[7]
	Language barriers[14,15]
	Medical illiteracy[14]
Environmental level	ED crowding[13,16]
	Inadequate post-ED care coordination[13,17]
	Frequent workflow interruptions[18]
	Time constraints[19]

Data from Refs.[8–19]

```
┌─────────────────────────────────────────────────────────────────┐
│                 1. Cultivating Safety Culture                     │
├─────────────────────────────────────────────────────────────────┤
│  Human Factors          Managerial Factors     Organizational Factors │
│  • Performance metrics   • Leadership support   •  Training in teamwork │
│  • Incentives            • Staff-led initiatives   and communication   │
│  • Education                                    •  Team communication   │
│                                                    techniques          │
│              Objectively measurement of patient safety                 │
└─────────────────────────────────────────────────────────────────┘
```

```
┌────────────────────────────────┐  ┌────────────────────────────────┐
│ 2. Implementing Processes to   │  │ 3. Creating Systems-based      │
│    Improve Patient Safety      │  │    Approaches to Patient Safety│
├────────────────────────────────┤  ├────────────────────────────────┤
│ • Safety event reporting        │  │ • Clinical practice guidelines  │
│   mechanism                     │  │ • Computerized physician order  │
│ • Morbidity & Mortality         │  │   entry                         │
│   conferences                   │  │ • Patient- and family-centered  │
│ • Patient safety walk-rounds    │  │   care                          │
└────────────────────────────────┘  └────────────────────────────────┘
```

Fig. 1. Framework for improving patient safety in the ED.

A recent systematic review of the literature on safety culture in the ED revealed 3 main factors influencing safety culture: (1) human factors, (2) managerial factors, and (3) organizational factors.[25] By breaking down how safety culture in the ED is shaped by these 3 factors, we can develop strategies to cultivate safety culture.

Human factors include perception of the ED staff toward patient safety and the systems in place to prevent errors.[25] It is thought that individual factors such as job title, motivation, and number of years at work affect safety culture in the ED.[25,26] An effective way to enhance the perception of patient safety at the individual level is to provide performance metrics and incentives related to patient safety for all clinical and administrative ED staff.[23] Combined with tracking safety metrics and incentivizing improvements in patient safety, ED staff should be provided with education on core patient safety concepts and topics at orientation and through ongoing safety conferences or grand rounds.[23,25]

Managerial factors include leadership support and prioritization of patient safety.[25] Selecting a discussion of patient safety issues as the first agenda item at the health care organization governance meetings and department leadership meetings is one way to highlight the organization's prioritization of patient safety.[23] However, a top-down approach may be insufficient in strengthening the organization's culture of safety. A study comparing 2 approaches to improving patient safety culture—one led by the ED physicians and another led by external facilitators from the hospital leadership—showed that the ED staff-led initiative correlated with higher patient safety rating, as well as staff engagement and support.[27]

Organizational factors include the formal processes and structures that are specifically designed to promote patient safety and prevent errors.[25] Training in teamwork and communication is one concrete way to improve patient safety culture in the ED. When the team leader models mutual respect and emphasizes psychological safety, team members report a safer environment for patients.[28,29] Communication within the ED can encompass many domains, including handoff communication between services, communication within the ED between teammates, and communication between patients and families.

Handoff has been a time that has been noted to be particularly high risk in emergency medicine.[30–32] System factors, such as those related to the clinical environment and the interprofessional relationships, as well as personal factors and training all likely play a role in exacerbating these challenges.[33] As such, opportunities to improve communication at the time of transition exist through both formal trainings and the new frameworks.[33] Among handoff communication frameworks that have been piloted in the ED are IPASS, the Targeted Solutions Tool, and the SBAR (situation, background, assessment, and recommendation).[34,35] These tools provide a framework for sharing critical information in a standard format (**Box 1**).[23,28,36] Interestingly, although many of the proposed communication tools stress the importance of verbal communication, there have also been exclusively electronic models of pass off proposed.[37] These asynchronous patient handoff processes are supported by structured electronic tools and offer a promising solution in the setting of ED overcrowding to ensure both efficiency and safety.

Communication between colleagues within the ED is also recognized as critical for patient safety. Examples of training curriculums that have been shown to be successful are Crisis Resource Management and Team Strategies and Tools to Enhance Performance and Patient Safety (TeamSTEPPS).[38] TeamSTEPPS used a 4-week training program designed to educate staff on how to communicate safety concerns and report errors and systems failures.[25,39,40] The program also focused on improving communication skills by facilitating group discussion with video vignettes to illustrate good communication skills and barriers to communication in the ED.[40] The implementation of TeamSTEPPS had a positive impact on perceived safety culture, decreased the number of communication-associated adverse events in the ED, and increased ED staff satisfaction and morale.[25,39,41] Another training program evaluated by Patterson and colleagues[42] incorporated a multidisciplinary simulation-based training module, which used video-based simulations to techniques to prevent medical errors, develop resilience and situational awareness, and master closed loop communication. This training module led to a statistically significant increase of patient safety knowledge among ED staff.[40,42] (see **Box 1**).

Patient safety culture should be measured objectively to assess its baseline and to monitor progress. One recommended tool for measuring patient safety in the ED is the validated Agency for Healthcare Research and Quality Survey on Patient Safety Culture.[43] The Agency for Healthcare Research and Quality Hospital Survey on Patient Safety Culture was developed using an iterative expert-based process with a review of the literature and other existing safety culture surveys.[44] Its survey items have demonstrated validity and reliability.[43] The survey includes a total of 51 items, measuring 12 composites that provides a level of detail that helps organizations

---

Box 1
SBAR (Situation, Background, Assessment, Recommendation) framework for communication between members of the health care team

S (Situation): Provide a concise statement of the problem

B (Background): Share pertinent information about the situation

A (Assessment): Articulate the analysis of the problem

R (Recommendation): Provide recommendations and actions required

Data from Institute for Healthcare Improvement (IHI). SBAR: Situation-Background-Assessment-Recommendation. Boston MA; 2017.

identify their areas of strengths and areas of improvement (**Box 2**). The survey is free and easily accessible, designed to be administered to all types of staff, including clinical and nonclinical staff in the ED. Health care organizations can voluntarily submit their survey data to the Agency for Healthcare Research and Quality Surveys on Patient Safety Culture Databases, which serves as central repositories and allows comparisons of survey results.

Implementing Processes to Improve Patient Safety

Safety culture is bolstered by nonpunitive processes that are designed to encourage approaching patient safety systematically. These processes are implemented to standardize continuous improvement in patient safety.

A well-studied process is a voluntary safety event reporting mechanism for staff to share their concerns.[45,46] The main purpose of safety event reporting is to learn from experience by analyzing adverse or near-miss events, leading to systematic change to prevent recurrences. Moreover, an aggregate voluntary reporting system can identify trends or recurrence of errors, thereby prompting the development of best practices to decrease future risks.[47] For a voluntary safety reporting system to be effective, it should be readily accessible and easy for staff to use to increase participation. An incident reporting program in the ED that implemented a campaign describing the importance of reporting while emphasizing the possibility of anonymous reporting, 24 hours/7 days a week open telephone reporting service, and feedback on analysis findings to all ED staff resulted in a statistically significant increase in reporting by the ED staff.[40,48] Feedback to the reporter is important for addressing concerns with potential solutions and for encouraging future reporting.[23] Developing a clearly stated and timely process for addressing safety event reports is important. In addition, a voluntary

---

Box 2
Twelve composites of the Agency for Healthcare Research and Quality Hospital Survey on Patient Safety Culture

1. Communication openness

2. Feedback and communication about error

3. Frequency of events reported

4. Hospital handoffs and transitions

5. Hospital management support for patient safety

6. Nonpunitive response to error

7. Organizational learning—continuous improvement

8. Overall perceptions of safety

9. Staffing

10. Supervisor/manager expectations and actions promoting patient safety

11. Teamwork across hospital units

12. Teamwork within units

Adapted from Sorra J, Gray L, Streagle S, et al. AHRQ Hospital Survey on Patient Safety Culture: User's Guide. Rockville, MD: Agency for Healthcare Research and Quality; January 2016. https://www.ahrq.gov/sites/default/files/wysiwyg/professionals/quality-patient-safety/patientsafetyculture/hospital/userguide/hospitalusersguide.pdf. Accessed September 29, 2019. With permission.

safety reporting system should prioritize the standardization of structured analysis and a nonpunitive peer review process of incident reports. A study that evaluated the effectiveness of a standardized, nonpunitive peer review process of incident reports showed that the monthly frequency of reporting increased over time, when compared with an analysis of incident reports by a single reviewer.[49] It is also recommended that information reported to internal and external review groups should not be discoverable in civil or legal actions.[23]

Morbidity and mortality conferences (M&M) are an important forum for formal debriefing and review of medical errors and quality issues in patient care in a systematic manner.[50] M&M also foster professional growth and responsibility while influencing practice change. M&M are perceived as important didactic tools in emergency medicine residency and are an Accreditation Council for Graduate Medical Education requirement.[51] A key to successful M&M is to create a supportive, inclusive environment that encourages opportunities to debrief challenging events.[44] Rather than focusing on individual performance and minimizing fear of blame or criticism, M&M should increase participants' comfort with openly discussing medical errors and brainstorm systematic approaches to decrease risks and avoid similar adverse events. Some of the elements of emergency medicine M&M that foster a strong culture of safety include the use of nonpunitive methods for case review, formal debriefing with staff involved in presented cases, conference formats that use anonymous case reporting, and follow-up of concrete actions taken to address systems issues.[52,53]

Implementation of patient safety walk-rounds (PSWs) has been shown to create a culture in which every team member feels comfortable to speak up about safety concerns. PSWs were originally developed to create open lines of communication about patient safety concerns and to help health care organization leaders to learn from front-line staff how to decrease the risk of medical errors.[54] On PSWs, clinical and operational leaders walks around care areas and talk directly with staff from all disciplines. In 1 study, PSWs implemented in the ED, performed by a physicians and 2 staff nurses, were found to be effective in increase in medication near-miss incident reports (44% increase) and in hand hygiene compliance within the ED (23% increase).[55] The experience of regular PSWs is thought to help bridge the gap between ED leadership and front-line staff perspectives on patient safety.[23,55]

Creating Systems-Based Approaches to Patient Safety

The last domain of the patient safety framework involves creating structural mechanisms to support a systems-based approaches to patient safety. This approach acknowledges that health care providers can make mistakes and their limitations should be accounted for in the design of the health care system.

To limit clinical practice variability in areas for which best practice has been defined on the basis of scientific evidence and expert consensus, the ED can develop and implement multidisciplinary evidence-based clinical practice guidelines for emergency care. The IOM defines clinical practice guidelines as "statements that include recommendations intended to optimize patient care that are informed by a systematic review of evidence and an assessment of the benefits and harms of alternative care options."[56] The implementation of clinical practice guidelines also can be tied with quality improvement initiatives as evidence-based recommendations form the basis of measurable standards for patient care. When considering the implementation of clinical practice guidelines, strategies to encourage the use of guidelines need to be considered. A review of 59 published evaluations of clinical practice guidelines showed that providing patient specific advice at the time of decision making, such as at the time of entering orders, is the most effective way to increase provider engagement and compliance.[57] Clinical practice guidelines must be reviewed and updated when new evidence suggests the need for consideration of clinically important recommendations.[56]

Electronic health records that integrate a computerized physician order entry (CPOE) system can also help to decrease errors. CPOE refers to the process of health care providers entering and sending patient care orders using a computer application.[58] A CPOE can serve as a platform that incorporates clinical practice guidelines. It can also provide timely clinical decision support that can provide treatment advice and automatically check for medication allergies, drug interactions, and other potential medical errors.[23,58] Studies examining the impact of CPOE implementation on patient safety showed that medication delivery error can be minimized by up to 80%.[59,60]

Last, the ED should prioritize integration of patient- and family-centered care. There are many barriers to forming partnerships with patients and families in the ED, such as the acute nature of medical needs, overcrowding, and the lack of a previous relationship between the patient and health care professionals. To overcome these myriad challenges, several training curriculums and core tenants of communication in the ED have been discussed in the literature that have focused on standardized introductions, fostering collaboration through empathy, acknowledgment of patients' emotions, reflective listening, and expectation setting.[61,62]

In addition, language barriers can prohibit health care providers from providing patient- and family-centered care while putting patients at a significantly increased risk for adverse events.[15] A study in 2014 found that the 3 common causes for medical errors related to language barriers were when (1) family members, friends, or nonqualified staff serve as interpreters, (2) cultural beliefs and traditions influence health care delivery, and (3) clinicians with insufficient language proficiency try to communicate without qualified interpreters.[59] Medication reconciliation, patient discharge, and informed consent were situations in which adverse events were mostly likely to occur owing to language barriers. The risk for adverse events can be decreased by providing patients and emergency care providers with timely access to qualified language translation support.[15]

SUMMARY

The ED is a complex environment, prone to risky decisions and medical errors, but staffed by dedicated professionals who strive to provide high quality care and improve patient safety. Since the IOM report in 1999, much has been learned about medical errors and how they are shaped by factors at the level of the provider, patient, and environment.

As more specialty boards incorporate quality improvement into maintenance of certification programs, health care professionals now understand and accept their role in proactively incorporating safety into their practice. The American Board of Emergency Medicine now requires clinically active American Board of Emergency Medicine-certified physicians to complete 2 "patient care practice improvement" activities every 10 years.[63] Furthermore, emergency physicians are uniquely positioned to analyze the challenges in patient safety throughout health care systems and to lead multidisciplinary efforts in patient safety improvement.

The proposed framework in this review provides a roadmap that stakeholders can use to develop strategic plans for improving safety culture and patient safety in the ED, and strategies for engaging health care professionals in patient safety culture. Through collaborative efforts and strategies that incorporate evidence-based practices, emergency physicians can take a leading role in improving patient care from the ED to the greater health care delivery system.

DISCLOSURE

The authors have nothing to disclose.

REFERENCES

1. Kohn L, Corrigan J, Donaldson M. To err is human: building a safer healthy system; National Academy Press. Washington, DC: 1999.
2. Brennan T, Leape L, Laird N, et al. Incidence of adverse events and negligence in hospitalized patients: results of the Harvard Medical Practice Study I. N Engl J Med 1999;324(6):370–6. https://doi.org/10.1136/qshc.2002.003822.
3. Thomas E, Studdert D, Burstin H, et al. Incidence and types of adverse events and negligent care in Utah and Colorado. Med Care 2000;38(3):261–71.
4. Hamedani A, Schuur J, Hobgood C, et al. Emergency medicine: clinical essentials. In: Adams J, Barton E, Collings J, et al, editors. 2nd edition. Philadelphia: Elsevier Inc; 2013. p. 1731–42.
5. Forster AJ, Rose NGW, Van Walraven C, et al. Adverse events following an emergency department visit. Qual Saf Health Care 2007;16(1):17–22. https://doi.org/10.1136/qshc.2005.017384.
6. Calder L, Foster A, Nelson M, et al. Adverse events among patients registered in high-acuity areas of the emergency department: a prospective cohort study. CJEM 2010;12(5):421–30.
7. Stang AS, Wingert AS, Hartling L, et al. Adverse events related to emergency department care: a systematic review. PLoS One 2013;8(9). https://doi.org/10.1371/journal.pone.0074214.
8. Gold DR, Rogacz S, Bock N, et al. Rotating shift work, sleep, and accidents related to sleepiness in hospital nurses. Am J Public Health 1992;82(7):1011–4.
9. Landrigan C, Rothschild J, Cronin J, et al. Effect of reducing interns' work hours on serious medical errors in intensive care units. N Engl J Med 2004;351(18):1838–48.
10. Rothschild J, Keohane C, Rogers S, et al. Risks of complications by attending physicians after performing nighttime procedures. JAMA 2009;302(14):1565–72.
11. Smits M, Groenewegen P, Timmermans D, et al. The nature and causes of unintended events reported at ten emergency departments. BMC Emerg Med 2009;9(1):16.
12. Joffe M. Emergency department provider fatigue and shift concerns. Clin Pediatr Emerg Med 2006;7:248–54.
13. Betsy Lehman Center for Patient Safety. Urgent matters: improving safety in Massachusetts Emergency Departments - A Betsy Lehman Center Expert Panel Report; Betsy Lehman Center for Patient Safety. Boston: 2019.
14. Sklar D, Crandall C. Perspectives on safety: what do we know about emergency department safety? Patient Safety Network, Agency of Healthcare Research and Quality. 2010. Available at: https://psnet.ahrq.gov/perspectives/perspective/88#tableback. Accessed September 26, 2019.
15. Cohen A, Rivara F, Marcuse E, et al. Are language barriers associated with serious medical events in hospitalized pediatric patients. Pediatrics 2005;116:575–9.
16. Hoot N, Aronsky D. Systematic review of emergency department crowding: causes, effects, and solutions. Ann Emerg Med 2008;52:126–36.

17. Vashi A, Rhodes K. "Sign Right Here and You're Good to Go": a content analysis of audiotaped emergency department discharge instructions. Ann Emerg Med 2011;57:315–22.

18. Chisolm C, Dornfeld A, Nelson D, et al. Work interrupted: a comparison of workplace interruptions in emergency departments and primary care offices. Ann Emerg Med 2001;38:146–51.

19. Fordyce J, Blank F, Pekow P, et al. Errors in a busy emergency department. Ann Emerg Med 2003;42(3):324–33.

20. World Health Organization. Conceptual Framework for the International Classification for Patient Safety; WHO. Geneva (Switzerland): 2009.

21. The Joint Commission on Accreditation of Healthcare Organizations. Comprehensive accreditation manual for hospitals; The Joint Commission. Oakbrook Terrace (IL): 2018.

22. Zohar D, Livne Y, Tenne-Gazit O, et al. Healthcare climate: a framework for measuring and improving patient safety. Crit Care Med 2007;35(5):1312–7.

23. Krug SE, Bojko T, Dolan MA, et al. Patient safety in the pediatric emergency care setting. Pediatrics 2007;120(6):1367–75. https://doi.org/10.1542/peds.2007-2902.

24. Bagian J. Patient safety: lessons learned. Pediatr Radiol 2006;36:287–90.

25. Alshyyab MA, FitzGerald G, Dingle K, et al. Developing a conceptual framework for patient safety culture in emergency department: a review of the literature. Int J Health Plann Manage 2019;34(1):42–55.

26. Tourani S, Hassani M, Ayoubian A, et al. Analyzing and prioritizing the dimensions of patient safety culture in emergency wards using the TOPSIS technique. Glob J Health Sci 2015;7(4):143–50.

27. Burström L, Letterstål A, Engström M, et al. The patient safety culture as perceived by staff at two different emergency departments before and after introducing a flow-oriented working model with team triage and lean principles: a repeated cross-sectional study. BMC Health Serv Res 2014;14(1):1–12.

28. Haig K, Sutton S, Whittington J. SBAR: a shared mental model for improving communication between clinicians. Jt Comm J Qual Patient Saf 2006;32:167–75.

29. Thomas E, Sexton J, Helmreich R. Translating teamwork behaviors from aviation to healthcare: development of behavioral markers for neonatal resuscitation. Qual Saf Health Care 2014;13(Suppl 1):1157–64.

30. Venkatesh A, Curley D, Chang Y, et al. Communication of vital signs at emergency department handoff: opportunities for improvement. Ann Emerg Med 2015;66(2):125–30.

31. Hilligoss B, Cohen M. The unappreciated challenges of between-unit handoffs: negotiating and coordinating across. Ann Emerg Med 2013;61(2):155–60.

32. Ye K, McD Taylor D, Knott J, et al. Handover in the emergency department: deficiencies and adverse effects. Emerg Med Australas 2007;19(5):433–41.

33. Olde Bekkink M, Farrell S, Takayesu J. Interprofessional communication in the emergency department: residents' perceptions and implications for medical education. Int J Med Educ 2018;25(9):262–70.

34. Heilman J, Flanigan M, Nelson A, et al. Adapting the I-PASS handoff program for emergency department inter-shift handoffs. West J Emerg Med 2016;17(6):756–61.

35. Benjamin M, Hargrave S, Nether K. Using the Targeted Solutions Tool® to Improve Emergency Department Handoffs in a Community Hospital. Jt Comm J Qual Patient Saf 2016;42(3):107–18.

36. Institute for Healthcare Improvement (IHI). SBAR: Situation-Background-Assessment-Recommendation. Boston: 2017.

37. Sanchez L, Chiu D, Nathanson L, et al. No title. J Emerg Med 2017;53(1):142–50.

38. Sweeney L, Warren O, Gardner L, et al. A simulation-based training program improves emergency department staff communication. Am J Med Qual 2014;29(2):115–23.

39. Jones F, Podila P, Powers C. Creating a culture of safety in the emergency department: the value of teamwork training. J Nurs Adm 2013;43:194–200.

40. Hesselink G, Berben S, Beune T, et al. Improving the governance of patient safety in emergency care: a systematic review of interventions. BMJ Open 2016;6(1). https://doi.org/10.1136/bmjopen-2015-009837.

41. Turner P. Implementation of TeamSTEPPS in the emergency department. Crit Care Nurs Q 2012;35(3):208–12.

42. Patterson M, Geis G, LeMaster T, et al. Impact of multidisciplinary simulation-based training on patient safety in a paediatric emergency department. BMJ Qual Saf 2013;22(5):383–93.

43. Agency for Healthcare Research and Quality (AHRQ). Hospital survey on patient safety culture: user's guide. Rockville, MD. 2018. Available at: https://www.ahrq.gov/sites/default/files/wysiwyg/professionals/quality-patient-safety/patientsafetyculture/hospital/userguide/hospitalusersguide.pdf. Accessed September 29, 2019.

44. Wittels K, Aaronson E, Dwyer R, et al. Emergency medicine morbidity and mortality conference and culture of safety: the resident perspective. AEM Educ Train 2017;1(3):191–9. https://doi.org/10.1002/aet2.10033.

45. Noord V, Bruijne D, Twisk J. The relationship between patient safety culture and the implementation of organizational patient safety defences at emergency departments. Int J Qual Health Care 2010;22(3):162–9.

46. Rigobello M, de Carvalho R, Guerreiro J, et al. The perception of the patient safety climate by professionals of the emergency department. Int Emerg Nurs 2017;33:1–6.

47. Lannon C, Coven B, Lane France F, et al. Principles of patient safety in pediatrics. Pediatrics 2001;107(6):1473–5.

48. Evans SM, Smith BJ, Esterman A, et al. Evaluation of an intervention aimed at improving voluntary incident reporting in hospitals. Qual Saf Health Care 2007;16(3):169–75.

49. Reznek M, Barton B. Improved incident reporting following the implementation of a standardized emergency department peer review process. Int J Qual Health Care 2014;26:278–86.

50. McVeigh T, Waters P, Murphy R, et al. Increasing reporting of adverse events to improve the educational value of the morbidity and mortality conference. J Am Coll Surg 2013;216:50–6.

51. Accreditation Council for Graduate Medical Education (ACGME). ACGME Program Requirements for Graduate Medical Education in Emergency Medicine. 2019. Available at: https://www.acgme.org/Portals/0/PFAssets/ProgramRequirements/110_EmergencyMedicine_2019_TCC.pdf?ver=2019-06-11-153018-223. Accessed October 9, 2019.

52. Sammer C, Lykens K, Singh K, et al. What is patient safety culture? A review of the literature. J Nurs Scholarsh 2010;42:156–65.

53. Jones K, Skinner A, Xu L, et al. The AHRQ Hospital Survey on patient safety culture : a tool to plan and evaluate patient safety programs; Agency for Healthcare Research and Quality. Rockville (MD): 2007.

54. Frankel A, Graydon-Baker E, Neppl C, et al. Patient safety leadership Walk-Rounds. Jt Comm J Qual Saf 2003;29:16–26.
55. Shaw K, Lavelle J, Crescenzo K, et al. Creating unit-based patient safety walk-rounds in a pediatric emergency department. Clin Pediatr Emerg Med 2006;7: 231–7.
56. Institute of Medicine (IOM). Clinical practice guidelines we can trust; National Academies Press. Washington, DC: 2011.
57. Vandvik P, Brandt L, Alonso-Coello P, et al. Creating clinical practice guidelines we can trust, use, and share: a new era is imminent. Chest 2013;144(2):381–9.
58. The Office of the National Coordinator for Health Information Technology. What is computerized provider order entry?. 2018. Available at: https://www.healthit.gov/faq/what-computerized-provider-order-entry. Accessed September 29, 2019.
59. Radley D, Wasserman M, Olsho L, et al. Reduction of medication errors in hospitals due to adoption of computerized provider order entry systems. J Am Med Inform Assoc 2013;6:1–7.
60. Bates D, Leape L, Cullen D, et al. Effect of computerized physician order entry and a team intervention on prevention of series medication errors. JAMA 1998; 6(15):1311–6.
61. Aaronson E, White B, Black L, et al. Training to improve communication quality: an efficient interdisciplinary experience for emergency department clinicians. Am J Med Qual 2019;34(3):260–5.
62. Rixon A, Rixon S, Addae-Bosomprah H, et al. Communication and influencing for ED professionals: a training programme developed in the emergency department for the emergency department. Emerg Med Australas 2016;28(4):404–11.
63. American Board of Emergency Medicine. Practice Improvement (PI). 2019. Available at: https://www.abem.org/public/stay-certified/improvement-in-medical-practice-(imp)/practice-improvement-(pi). Accessed October 11, 2019.

Optimizing Patient Experience in the Emergency Department

Jonathan D. Sonis, MD, MHCM*, Benjamin A. White, MD

KEYWORDS

- Patient experience • Satisfaction • Communication • Empathy • Logic modeling
- PFAC • Discharge

KEY POINTS

- Despite many experience challenges intrinsic to the emergency department (ED) care model, the ED represents a unique opportunity to create a positive first impression of a hospital or health system for patients and their families.
- Improved ED patient experience and, in particular, staff-patient communication have important implications for patient health outcomes, staff satisfaction, and risk management.
- Although perceived wait times are a major driver of ED patient experience, other factors, including perceived empathy and staff-patient communication, are greater contributors to overall satisfaction.
- Given the complexity of ED patient experience, consider logic modeling to develop a framework of the contexts, service delivery factors, and desired outcomes to guide improvement initiatives.
- Establishing formal communication training programs, ED patient call-back systems, and patient and family advisory councils are high-yield interventions to optimize ED patient experience.

BACKGROUND

As an emergency department (ED) visit often represents a patient's initial encounter with a health care system, it is a unique opportunity to establish a positive first impression. However, several factors intrinsic to the ED care model and environment make it a challenging area for improving the patient experience, including a lack of preexisting relationships among providers, staff, and patients; unpredictable waits; overcrowding; and limited privacy.[1–3]

Drs J.D. Sonis and B.A. White have no commercial or financial conflicts of interest.
Department of Emergency Medicine, Massachusetts General Hospital, Harvard Medical School, 55 Fruit Street, Founders 850, Boston, MA 02114, USA
* Corresponding author.
E-mail address: Sonis@MGH.HARVARD.EDU

Emerg Med Clin N Am 38 (2020) 705–713
https://doi.org/10.1016/j.emc.2020.04.008
0733-8627/20/© 2020 Elsevier Inc. All rights reserved.
emed.theclinics.com

Despite these challenges, patient experience has recently been a growing area of focus for leaders at the ED, hospital, and health care system levels, especially given data suggesting that poor ED experiences can drive lower ratings of inpatient experience.[4,5] Not only do departmental efforts on patient experience lead to improvement in survey scores of patient experience, recent literature suggests that enhancing the ED patient experience also reduces risk management episodes, improves staff satisfaction (and subsequently decreases provider burnout), and increases revenue.[1,6–11] Perhaps most importantly, improvements in ED patient experience, and, particularly, provider and staff-patient communication, may lead to increased compliance with plans of care, and ultimately, improved objective health outcomes.[12,13]

Furthering the timeliness of a focus on the ED patient experience, the ongoing development of the Centers for Medicare and Medicaid Services (CMS) Emergency Department Patient Experience of Care (EDPEC) survey suggests that ED patient-reported experience data will soon be publicly reported, much like that of the Hospital Consumer Assessment of Healthcare Providers and Systems (HCAHPS) survey.[14–16] In addition, assuming that EDPEC will follow a similar incentive and penalty program to that of HCAHPS, Medicare reimbursement may soon be tied to total performance on the EDPEC survey.

CONTRIBUTING FACTORS

Although wait times are often cited as a critical driver of the ED patient experience, recent literature suggests that the key determinants are the quality of staff-patient communication, patients' perception of staff empathy and compassion, the quality of pain management, and patients' perception of technical competence.[1,3,17] Factors including the environment of care, privacy, cleanliness, noise, and food availability, among others, are likely less critical in forming patients' overall perception.[1,3]

Drivers of the Emergency Department Patient Experience

- Staff-patient communication
- Staff empathy and compassion
- Patient expectations
- Actual and perceived wait times/timeliness of care
- Environment of care/cleanliness
- Pain control and comfort
- Perceived staff technical skill and competence
- Convenience factors (ie, food availability, parking)

Although each of these have been studied extensively over the past decade, the relative importance of each of these themes has not been clearly established.[1,2]

Through logic modeling, a conceptual framework can be developed to allow for the visualization of the relationships between preexisting realities (ie, overcrowding), potential interventions, and expected outcomes related to themes within the ED patient experience[18,19] (Fig. 1).

HIGH-YIELD INTERVENTIONS

Given the aforementioned challenges in creating excellence in the ED patient experience, a focus on high-yield interventions that aim at factors amenable to rapid, measurable improvement is critical. Potential interventions can be categorized into 3 major themes: Systems Factors, Patient Factors, and Staff Factors. Although wait

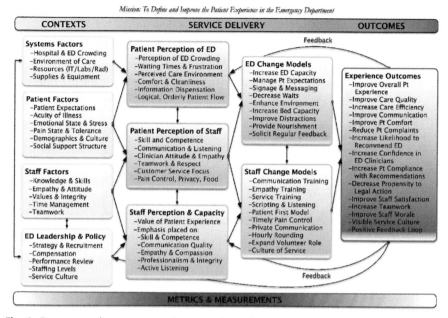

Fig. 1. Emergency department patient experience logic model.

and throughput times are significant drivers of the ED patient experience, these are discussed elsewhere and will not be a focus of this section.

Systems Factors

- Improve the Environment of CareED patients' perception of the quality of the medical care received is impacted by the environment in which it is received. Although a minimum of thorough cleaning of each ED bay between patient visits is necessary, a rotating deep cleaning schedule, by which each area of the ED is closed allowing for more intensive cleaning (eg, floor polishing, washing walls) can improve both appearance and infection control.Providing ED care in private bays, when possible, serves to enhance patients' perception of privacy and has the additional benefit of reducing rates of infection.[2] When private bays are impractical, using portable privacy screens for patients cared for in hallways, dedicated private conversation spaces so that sensitive discussions do not take place in public spaces, and reminding patients that their privacy is valued (ie, "I am going to close this curtain to give us some privacy") all serve to enhance the perception of privacy.Last, to maintain a professional environment, consider limiting wall postings throughout the ED to those that are directed toward patients and their families.
- Formalize Discharge TeachingCommunication with patients and their families at the time of discharge is critical in creating a positive last impression of their ED visit. When focused and clear, discharge teaching may have the added benefits of improving follow-up compliance and decreasing unnecessary revisits.[20]The ED discharge communication process should be formalized so that it is clear which staff member is responsible for delivering instructions and ensuring that all of a patient's questions have been addressed. A patient discharge checklist

can be used to empower patients to take ownership of their discharge plan, and safeguard against missed steps in the process (**Fig. 2**).

Patient Factors

- Provide Adequate NourishmentAlthough EDs do not require luxurious dining options, in light of the prolonged times that patients may spend in the ED, providing adequate food to patients is vital to allow them to participate in their care and

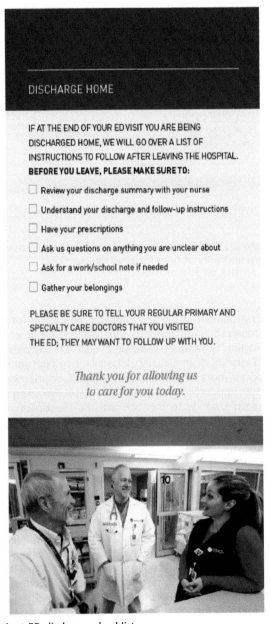

Fig. 2. Sample patient ED discharge checklist.

comprehend management decisions. Patients who are kept "NPO" (nothing by mouth) without medical necessity are more likely to become impulsive or aggressive toward staff and other patients and, given accompanying psychological changes, may be unable to appreciate positive aspects of their ED patient experience.[21] If no 24-hour-per-day food service is available, readily accessible vending machines, from which patients or family members can purchase a variety of food and beverage options, serves to mitigate this risk.

- Enhance Patient ComfortAlthough overcrowding, privacy limitations, and other factors create comfort challenges for ED patients, simple low-resource gestures such as the offering of a warm blanket or pillow can substantially improve patients' perception of compassion.[11]
- Focus on PerceptionAlthough research demonstrates that wait times are an important contributor to ED patient experience, perceived waiting times are stronger determinants of patient experience than actual waiting times.[11,22,23] Given this, distractions such as mobile device charging stations, welcome materials or signage to orient patients and their families to the ED, and accessible Web-based health promotion tools (ie, smoking cessation or healthy diet resources) may improve patient experience through decreasing perceived wait times. Although limited research suggests that isolated interventions like providing bedside personal televisions has little effect on the overall ED patient experience, a comprehensive approach to improving perceptions of wait times may be of greater benefit.[24]
- Provide Timely Acknowledgment of PainMuch like patients who have not received adequate nourishment, those who are in significant pain are not likely to focus on positive aspects of their ED experience, and more importantly, they cannot adequately engage in care decisions or comprehend management plans. To avoid delays in pain medication administration, a management pathway beginning at triage can expedite appropriate analgesia. This intervention, by which patients reporting a given pain score on initial evaluation trigger a process by which standardized analgesic orders are placed, serves not only to improve patient experience, but also to decrease the likelihood of patients leaving without being seen by a provider.[1,25,26] Importantly, in creating such a pathway, emphasis must be placed on ensuring that all patients, regardless of race, ethnicity, age, or sex, are treated equally, as extensive evidence exists suggesting under or delayed treatment of pain in minority and female patients.[27–29]

Staff Factors

- Teach a Communication ToolboxAs discussed more extensively in *Best Practices in Patient Safety and Communication*, staff-patient communication is among the most significant drivers of the ED patient experience.[1,3,11] Specific aspects of provider or staff-patient communication, including acknowledging all visitors with the patient, introducing all members of the care team, and providing realistic estimates of wait times, are particularly high-yield. Tools such as the Studer Group's AIDET (Acknowledge, Introduce, Duration, Explanation, Thank You) or EMPATHY (Eye contact, Muscles of facial expression, Posture, Affect, Tone of voice, Hearing the whole patient, Your response) can be helpful reminders for staff to be mindful of their communication techniques.[30,31]
- Sit DownThe simple act of providers sitting down while conducting patient encounters has dramatic effects on patients' impressions of their caregivers and their perception of time spent at the bedside. Research suggests that providers

who sit at the bedside may require less time than those who stand.[32] Reduce the burden of sitting by ensuring that every ED bay is equipped with a stool or folding chair that is marked clearly to be used for providers only.

EFFECTING CHANGE

ED providers want to treat patients and their families well, but face significant challenges in their attempts to provide an excellent patient experience given the factors intrinsic to ED care listed previously, as well as production pressure, and measureable decreases in their experience of compassion over time (referred to in some sources as "compassion fatigue").[33,34] Critical to providing an excellent ED patient experience is creating a departmental culture in which all staff value its importance, and feel empowered to take steps to improve individual patients' experiences. Although the development of a reward program (ie, public recognition or financial incentives) for those who excel in discrete and measurable patient experience standards may be beneficial, all ED staff need to be equipped with the necessary skills and tools to succeed in this realm.

To address the need for formal training for ED staff, particularly regarding communication techniques, a variety of interventions have been successful, leading not only to improved patient experience but also decreased staff burnout.[35,36] Hands-on programs in which ED staff practice specific communication skills related to expectation setting, conflict resolution, acknowledgment of patient concerns, and staff-patient collaboration, may be particularly high-yield in promoting culture change.[37]

PATIENT PERSPECTIVES
Patient and Family Advisory Council

Obtaining useful data about the drivers of the ED patient experience and the perspectives of a particular ED's patients are difficult, and can frustrate traditional data-gathering methods.[38] Although many EDs use a post-visit survey tool to better understand patient experiences, survey data may be limited by poor response rates and nonresponse bias.[39] Further, ED leadership rarely has the opportunity to delve into responses to gain a deeper understanding of patients' perspectives or ideas.

To increase direct patient input into improving the ED patient experience, an ED Patient and Family Advisory Council (PFAC) may be developed. Through the formation of a group of dedicated patients, family members, and selected ED clinical and administrative staff, an ED PFAC can serve multiple purposes[40]:

1. Gain unique insight into the existing ED patient experience.
2. Discover novel patient-driven approaches to improving the ED patient experience.
3. Receive feedback on existing initiatives, focusing efforts and resources.
4. Strengthen relationships with community members who have demonstrated interest in ED patient experience improvement (or concerns about the existing experience).

Emergency Department Patient Call-Back Program

A call-back program, through which patients who were discharged from the ED are contacted by phone by a trained staff member (ie, a nurse or advanced practice provider) following discharge, is another critical method of obtaining patient experience feedback. Unlike survey administration, which may be delayed several weeks following the ED visit, patient call-backs should be conducted within a short time from discharge, capturing patients' feedback while it is still fresh. In addition, by allowing for open-ended responses, feedback is not limited to numeric ratings.

The development of a formal ED patient call-back program serves 3 main goals:

1. Improve perception of the ED visit and significantly increase ratings of the ED experience.[41,42]
2. Reinforce discharge planning, including follow-up instructions and therapy compliance.[42]
3. Identify clinical deterioration or other issues warranting return to the ED.[42]

SUMMARY

Patient experience in the ED is a growing area of focus for departmental, hospital, and health care system leaders. With the ongoing development and upcoming release of the Centers for Medicare and Medicaid Services EDPEC survey, this emphasis will only increase. Although a variety of factors including the environment of care and adequacy and timeliness of pain control contribute to the ED patient experience, data suggest that staff-patient communication and, specifically, the expression of compassion and empathy, is of particular importance. Notably, although wait and throughput times affect ED patient experience, perceived wait times, as opposed to actual wait times, have a larger effect. Given these findings, initiatives to improve ED patient experience should focus on staff-provider communication techniques, the expression of empathy, and the reduction of perceived waits.

REFERENCES

1. Welch SJ. Twenty years of patient satisfaction research applied to the emergency department: a qualitative review. Am J Med Qual 2010;25(1):64–72.
2. Taylor C, Benger JR. Patient satisfaction in emergency medicine. Emerg Med J 2004;21(5):528–32.
3. Sonis JD, Aaronson EL, Lee RY, et al. Emergency department patient experience: a systematic review of the literature. J Patient Exp 2018;5(2):101–6.
4. Increasing value in the emergency department: using data to drive improvement. South Bend (IN): Press Ganey; 2015.
5. Wolf JA, NV, Marshburn D, et al. Defining patient experience. Patient Experience J 2014;1(1).
6. Hickson GB, Federspiel CF, Pichert JW, et al. Patient complaints and malpractice risk. JAMA 2002;287(22):2951–7.
7. Stelfox HT, Gandhi TK, Orav EJ, et al. The relation of patient satisfaction with complaints against physicians and malpractice lawsuits. Am J Med 2005;118(10): 1126–33.
8. Lu DW, Dresden S, McCloskey C, et al. Impact of burnout on self-reported patient care among emergency physicians. West J Emerg Med 2015;16(7):996–1001.
9. Lee T. Physician burnout and patient experience: flip sides of the same coin. Catalyst 2016.
10. Wright KB. A communication competence approach to healthcare worker conflict, job stress, job burnout, and job satisfaction. J Healthc Qual 2011;33(2):7–14.
11. Boudreaux ED, O'Hea EL. Patient satisfaction in the Emergency Department: a review of the literature and implications for practice. J Emerg Med 2004;26(1): 13–26.

12. Chang JT, Hays RD, Shekelle PG, et al. Patients' global ratings of their health care are not associated with the technical quality of their care. Ann Intern Med 2006; 144(9):665–72.

13. Levinson W, Lesser CS, Epstein RM. Developing physician communication skills for patient-centered care. Health Aff (Millwood) 2010;29(7):1310–8.

14. Emergency Department Patient Experiences with Care (EDPEC) Survey. Available at: https://www.cms.gov/Research-Statistics-Data-and-Systems/Research/CAHPS/ed.html. Accessed February 12, 2019.

15. Giordano LA, Elliott MN, Goldstein E, et al. Development, implementation, and public reporting of the HCAHPS survey. Med Care Res Rev 2010;67(1):27–37.

16. HCAHPS Hospital Consumer Assessment of Healthcare Providers and Systems. Centers for Medicare & Medicaid Services. Available at: http://www.hcahpsonline.org. Accessed February 12, 2019.

17. Aaronson EL, Mort E, Sonis JD, et al. Overall emergency department rating: identifying the factors that matter most to patient experience. J Healthc Qual 2018; 40(6):367–76.

18. Clapham K, Manning C, Williams K, et al. Using a logic model to evaluate the Kids Together early education inclusion program for children with disabilities and additional needs. Eval Program Plann 2017;61:96–105.

19. Sonis JD, Aaronson EL, Castagna A, et al. A conceptual model for emergency department patient experience. J Patient Exp 2019;6(3):173–8.

20. McCarthy DM, Engel KG, Buckley BA, et al. Emergency department discharge instructions: lessons learned through developing new patient education materials. Emerg Med Int 2012;2012:306859.

21. Fessler DM. The implications of starvation induced psychological changes for the ethical treatment of hunger strikers. J Med Ethics 2003;29(4):243–7.

22. Hedges JR, Trout A, Magnusson AR. Satisfied patients exiting the emergency department (SPEED) study. Acad Emerg Med 2002;9(1):15–21.

23. Thompson DA, Yarnold PR, Williams DR, et al. Effects of actual waiting time, perceived waiting time, information delivery, and expressive quality on patient satisfaction in the emergency department. Ann Emerg Med 1996;28(6):657–65.

24. Singer AJ, Sanders BT, Kowalska A, et al. The effect of introducing bedside TV sets on patient satisfaction in the ED. Am J Emerg Med 2000;18(1):119–20.

25. Arendt KW, Sadosty AT, Weaver AL, et al. The left-without-being-seen patients: what would keep them from leaving? Ann Emerg Med 2003;42(3):317–23.

26. Yanuka M, Soffer D, Halpern P. An interventional study to improve the quality of analgesia in the emergency department. CJEM 2008;10(5):435–9.

27. Todd KH. Pain assessment and ethnicity. Ann Emerg Med 1996;27(4):421–3.

28. Tanabe P, Myers R, Zosel A, et al. Emergency department management of acute pain episodes in sickle cell disease. Acad Emerg Med 2007;14(5):419–25.

29. Todd KH, Samaroo N, Hoffman JR. Ethnicity as a risk factor for inadequate emergency department analgesia. JAMA 1993;269(12):1537–9.

30. Riess H, Kraft-Todd G. E.M.P.A.T.H.Y.: a tool to enhance nonverbal communication between clinicians and their patients. Acad Med 2014;89(8):1108–12.

31. Barber S. Patient care in decline: AIDET as a tool for improvement. Radiol Technol 2018;89(4):419–21.

32. Swayden KJ, Anderson KK, Connelly LM, et al. Effect of sitting vs. standing on perception of provider time at bedside: a pilot study. Patient Educ Couns 2012; 86(2):166–71.

33. Chen D, Lew R, Hershman W, et al. A cross-sectional measurement of medical student empathy. J Gen Intern Med 2007;22(10):1434–8.

34. Mandel ED, Schweinle WE. A study of empathy decline in physician assistant students at completion of first didactic year. J Physician Assist Educ 2012;23(4): 16–24.
35. Boissy AWA, Bokar D, Karafa M, et al. Communication skills training for physicians improves patient satisfaction. J Gen Intern Med 2016;31:755–61.
36. Bonvicini KA, Perlin MJ, Bylund CL, et al. Impact of communication training on physician expression of empathy in patient encounters. Patient Educ Couns 2009;75(1):3–10.
37. Aaronson EL, White BA, Black L, et al. Training to improve communication quality: an efficient interdisciplinary experience for emergency department clinicians. Am J Med Qual 2019;34(3):260–5.
38. Working with patients and families as advisors. AHRQ. Available at: https://www.ahrq. gov/sites/default/files/wysiwyg/professionals/systems/hospital/engagingfamilies/strategy1/ Strat1_Implement_Hndbook_508_v2.pdf. Accessed February 12, 2019.
39. Tyser AR, Abtahi AM, McFadden M, et al. Evidence of non-response bias in the Press-Ganey patient satisfaction survey. BMC Health Serv Res 2016;16(a):350.
40. Sonis JD, Hughes M, Kraus C, et al. Getting off the ground: developing an ED patient and family advocacy council to improve patient experience. In: Common sense. American Academy of Emergency Medicine; 2019. Available at: https:// www.aaem.org/resources/publications/common-sense/issues/featured-articles/ getting-off-the-ground-developing-an-ed-patient-and-family-advocacy-council-to-improve-patient-experience.
41. Guss DA, Gray S, Castillo EM. The impact of patient telephone call after discharge on likelihood to recommend in an academic emergency department. J Emerg Med 2014;46(4):560–6.
42. Shesser R, Smith M, Adams S, et al. The effectiveness of an organized emergency department follow-up system. Ann Emerg Med 1986;15(8):911–5.

Management of the Academic Emergency Department

Deborah Vinton, MD, MBA[a],*, Leon D. Sanchez, MD, MPH[b]

KEYWORDS

- Operations • Process improvement • Academic medical centers • Leadership
- Quality management

KEY POINTS

- Academic EDs play a critical role in educating future ED physicians, providing novel emergent care, and conducting research.
- Academic EDs face enormous challenges because of the decline of governmental funding for research and education and shifting payment models that emphasize efficiency and value.
- Facing such challenges, leadership within academic EDs must engage in continuous process improvement efforts to deliver more efficient care, conduct operational research, and design staffing models that promote education and account for the variability in trainee productivity.
- By improving operational efficiency and the quality of patient care, academic EDs can better contribute to national efforts that may make health care more affordable and become as clinically efficient as possible, while also supporting a complex tripartite academic mission.

INTRODUCTION

Academic emergency departments (EDs), defined as academic-affiliated EDs that engage in on-site resident education with core faculty attending supervision, play a vital role in the provision of emergency care and contributing to the training of resident physicians. Academic EDs also have a major role in generating innovations and discoveries through clinical research within US academic medical centers (AMCs).[1,2] Academic EDs need to deliver high-value care that is high in quality and efficiency. They can face increased challenges when initiating operational process improvement

[a] Department of Emergency Medicine, University of Virginia Health System, PO Box 800699, Charlottesville, VA 22908-0699, USA; [b] Department of Emergency Medicine, Beth Israel Deaconess Medical Center, Boston, MA, USA
* Corresponding author.
E-mail address: dv9j@hscmail.mcc.virginia.edu

Emerg Med Clin N Am 38 (2020) 715–727
https://doi.org/10.1016/j.emc.2020.03.006
0733-8627/20/© 2020 Elsevier Inc. All rights reserved.

efforts because of the medical complexity of patients, the academic culture within AMCs, and the variability in productivity and specialty training of trainees. This article explores the characteristics shared by academic EDs, how to implement process improvement initiatives, the impact that trainees have on ED operations, and how to best promote operational research so as to optimize ED operations within an academic setting.

CHARACTERIZATION OF ACADEMIC EMERGENCY DEPARTMENTS: PATIENT CARE AND REIMBURSEMENTS

AMCs and academic EDs have a large economic impact within the United States, accounting for approximately $562 billion annually, or 3.1% of the gross domestic product, according to the Association of American Medical Colleges.[3,4] In addition to providing their surrounding communities with high-quality medical care, AMCs create jobs, support medical research and scientific advancements, contribute to new business development, and educate the nation's health care workforce. Academic EDs often provide critical roles as trauma centers and leadership in disaster preparedness **(Fig. 1)**.[5] AMCs collectively graduate more than 19,000 physicians each year and conduct the most basic, clinical, and health services research.[6]

Academic EDs comprise only 5% of total EDs in the United States and have unique challenges and opportunities related to their tripartite mission of clinical operations, education, and research **(Fig. 2)**. They tend to be concentrated in large hospitals that can support their training mission while serving as tertiary care centers and safety nets for their surrounding communities. Within the greater AMC, academic EDs play a unique role in which they provide care for the sickest patients and a large share of low-income individuals who qualify for charity care and Medicaid beneficiaries.[7,8] As a result, AMCs and academic EDs provide a disproportionate amount of care for highly acute patients and disadvantaged patients. Some of the costs of uncompensated care may be defrayed by Medicare disproportionate share hospital payments, Medicaid disproportionate share hospital payments, and payments for

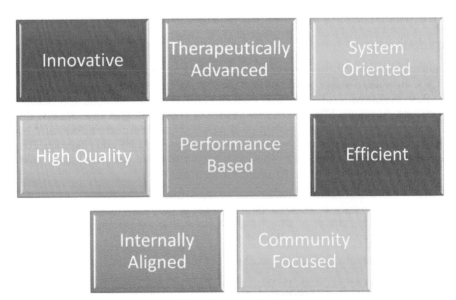

Fig. 1. Characteristics of a successful academic medical center.

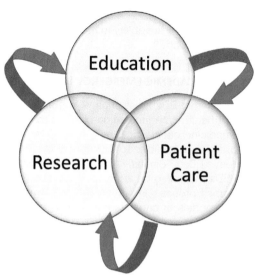

Fig. 2. AMC tripartite mission.

undocumented immigrants. However, this leaves academic EDs extremely vulnerable to changes in government payment policies and reductions in Centers for Medicare and Medicaid Services reimbursements.[9]

The distinct role that academic EDs play in providing care for complex patients and the increases in ED visits in the wake of Medicaid expansion in many states presents many academic EDs with programmatic and operational challenges.[10,11] Recent publications suggest that within academic EDs, the annual patient census increased 13.4% over a 5-year period ending in 2016, with 80% of the sites surveyed experiencing growth over the survey period.[12] Acuity and severity as measured by the Emergency Severity Index level 1 and 2 also increased in academic EDs during the study. Large-volume EDs experienced an increase in admissions of more than 15%, likely related to a surge in overall patient volumes. Emergency medical service arrivals increased by 7.3%, with admission rates from emergency medical service arrivals remaining stable. As volumes increased, left without being seen rates decreased by 19.5%, but total walk-outs, including left without being discharged or patients who left the ED against medical advice, did not. These data suggest that these centers are seeing increases in patient volume, acuity, and underlying illness severity, all of which require an increased number of resources. These trends are essential for the operational leaders within academic EDs to take into account when projecting staffing and resource needs.[13]

Simultaneously, many of these facilities face a resource crunch because of a decline of governmental funding for research and education while payment models shift to emphasize operational efficiency and value.[14] To realize their tripartite mission while ensuring financial viability, academic EDs must strive to improve efficiency, cost, and patient satisfaction while maintaining the resources to continue developing trainees and engaging in clinical research. ED operational leadership within academic centers must seek to deliver appropriate, high-quality care with excellent outcomes, efficient delivery, convenience, and low cost. This is especially critical as the focus of health care delivery shifts to incentivize the quality of care and enhancing value to the customer.[15–17] Academic EDs, just as in the community, will fall under the scrutiny of policymakers, payers, and patients who will have the expectation that EDs publish performance data and have the ability to meaningfully respond to any critique of ED services or ongoing research.[15]

PROCESS IMPROVEMENT IN ACADEMIC EMERGENCY DEPARTMENTS

Like community EDs, academic EDs must engage in continuous process improvement. The drive to adopt health care innovations in ED practice, such as new fast-track models and telemedicine capabilities, has to be carefully tempered with the transferability of such practices or policies to the high-acuity and low-resource patient population within academic EDs.[18] Similarly, the unique faculty and practice environment within academic EDs must also be addressed, because the culture of an academic facility may hamper process improvement and create unique challenges when implementing new models of care. Academic EDs also need to explore new models of training to ensure residency programs are educating new physicians who are well-versed in clinical techniques and care models that work best as the landscape for health care continues to change.

Organizational transformation focusing on operational efficiency is extremely challenging in an academic ED setting. Academic EDs are often not designed for high-speed change because of the complicated missions, governance structures, and underlying faculty dynamics.[19] Faculty are often motivated by such factors as research, education, and intellectual curiosity rather than improving metrics, and operational concerns can run contrary to these other priorities. Within AMCs, the hierarchical structure may not necessarily favor individual administrators championing process improvement. Furthermore, the presence of multiple cultural hierarchies, including researchers, undergraduate and graduate medical educators, and clinical and educational nursing leaders, can make quality improvement efforts within academic EDs be orders of magnitude harder than in other health care settings. As a result, some AMCs are slow to adopt innovative care practices, and often are less efficient in the delivery of care compared with competing community EDs.

Given these challenges, several measures can be taken to more successfully implement process improvement projects to enhance efficiency within academic EDs. Successful tactics include engaging expert clinicians across multiple subspecialties to reach consensus and develop protocols to better standardize clinical care and reduce variability within clinical practice. Given faculty interests and diverging roles in academic departments, physician participants in process improvement efforts must also be provided with sufficient time free from competing academic responsibilities to engage in projects, and sufficient departmental resources must be allocated to the project in advance to promote faculty engagement.[20] Although divergent philosophies on patient care may still hamper efforts to improve quality and lower health care costs, inviting nonadministrative physicians to contribute to the decision-making process and serve as champions for change is key to improving the quality and value of care within the ED. Leadership within AMCs and academic EDs must demonstrate a high degree of commitment to proposed improvement initiatives with a clear set of objectives that are data-driven. For academic faculty to adopt operational changes, there must also be an emphasis on empirical data with clear quality improvement efforts that are not only specific to clinical care but to the AMC teaching mission as well.

In addition to using the aforementioned strategies to engage academic faculty in process improvement efforts, multiple methodologies exist to promote operational excellence and improve the quality of patient care within an academic ED. Many academic institutions are turning to Lean methodology, which has been effective in other sectors to streamline processes and achieve excellent results in a cost-effective manner. Lean's core principle is that each process needs to add value as defined by the patient, and any step that fails to add value is deemed "waste." The aims of Lean methodology are to therefore eliminate waste to improve processes and ensure that all steps within the patient care process are truly "value added" steps (**Fig. 3**).[21–23] Although Lean methodology is an excellent technique to improve efficiency, in the academic ED setting, the educational mission of the institution must be considered when implementing Lean techniques. Although certain processes may not add value directly to the patient, a variety of redundant processes may enhance education and promote the training of medical students, residents, and fellows practicing within the ED.[24] Likewise, processes' impact on clinical research must be taken into account when considering any analysis or improvement. Engaging teaching faculty and researchers early in the course of process improvement efforts ensures that these complex interests are considered and can help to build support for decisions that change physician workflow or models of care.

Similar to Lean methodologies, Six Sigma is a prominent methodology within the manufacturing sector and is driving process improvement and ultimately patient care within many academic settings.[25] The emphasis of Six Sigma is on setting high objectives, collection of data, and analysis of results to reduce defects within the current operational processes.[26] Six Sigma emphasizes the need to measure defects so that a system can find ways to eliminate those defects and refine operations and move closer to "perfection."[27] Using the DMAIC method (Define, Measure, Analyze, Improve, Control) to uncover deviations and solve existing problems, Six Sigma at its core uses data and statistics to draw conclusions and optimize health care processes (**Box 1**).[28] In academic EDs, many of the processes involved in providing patient care are highly repeatable and lend themselves to the application of Six Sigma principles. Six Sigma has a tight focus on finding the voice of the customer, which is particularly complex in academic settings because the customers may be patients, trainees, or researchers, all of whom have different needs. Six Sigma's emphasis on analytical data to drive process improvement lends itself to the academic setting and as long as champions of process improvement efforts focus on highlighting how efforts will lead to improvement in the quality and safety of patient care, this strategy can yield useful results.

Process Activity	Lean
Value Added Activity	⬆ Optimize
Essential Non-Value Add Activity	⬌ Minimize
Non-Value Add Activity	⬇ Eliminate

Fig. 3. Three types of Lean process activities.

> **Box 1**
> **Six sigma DMAIC methodology**
>
> 1. Define the problem statement then clarify scope and measurable goals
> 2. Measure process performance and identify performance gaps
> 3. Analyze the data and determine root cause of defects and waste
> 4. Improve the process by addressing and eliminating root causes
> 5. Control and maintain the improved process by implementing error proofing measures and monitoring performance

The human-centered process innovation methodology of Design Thinking also offers an innovative approach to problem solving within academic EDs and is ideal for solving abstract problems that lack concrete solutions related to patient care. Widely used in business and technology, the methodology is now being adopted in the health care setting. Design Thinking is an innovation process that prioritizes deep empathy for end-user needs to understand complex, system-wide problems and develop more effective solutions.[29,30] To do so, Design Thinking takes health care teams through five steps: (1) empathize, (2) define, (3) ideate, (4) prototype, and (5) test (**Fig. 4**). Throughout these steps, the methodology focuses on brainstorming, user needs, and collaboration, making it ideally suited for academic settings where engaging a multidisciplinary team of academicians is critical to ensure the success of the project.[31] Given this methodology's innovative and agile approach to process improvement, many AMCs are creating Design Thinking curricula to encourage its use. Although likely not an ideal method to address problems that are well understood or have a limited set of possible solutions, Design Thinking holds great promise for many patient-centered initiatives within the academic setting.

When considering introducing any of these process improvement methodologies, academic EDs should offer training to front-line staff, including nurses, physicians, and administrators, all of whom can then apply the tools and then champion subsequent improvement while remaining in their current roles.[32] Involving experts from areas affected by a process improvement project is also important for buy-in; if a project involves improving care for patients with stroke admitted from the ED, involve the neurologists who will be admitting the patient. Projects' improvements to patient safety and quality of care should be emphasized, rather than potential financial savings.

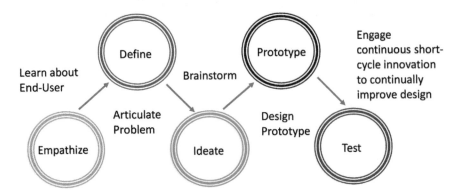

Fig. 4. Design Thinking workflow process.

IMPACT OF TRAINEES ON OPERATIONS IN ACADEMIC EMERGENCY DEPARTMENTS

Although engaging academic ED faculty in improvement efforts and operationalizing those efforts is challenging, the constant turnover of trainees, variability in trainees' skills sets and productivity, and the unique scheduling constraints within academic departments also creates hurdles to improving efficiency and quality. Within academic EDs many providers are resident physicians. Some of these may be rotators from other services and only work in the ED for a few weeks a year or over the total duration of their training. Every June, the most senior and experienced class of emergency medicine (EM) residents graduate and a new group of intern residents enter the ED workforce.[33] For many EDs, this "July effect" represents a sharp transition away from maximum efficiency.[34–36] This collective turnover of resident trainees increases operational costs and indirect costs, such as the loss of organizational knowledge, and has the potential to reduce productivity, lowers patient satisfaction, and poses a constant risk to the quality of care delivered in the ED.[37–39]

The monthly and annual turnover of residents results in known and unavoidable recurring challenges in staffing and efficiency. Although research suggests that no significant differences in ED patient length of stay clearly occur in July relative to other months, residents nevertheless have longer door-to-doctor times and times to disposition at the beginning of the academic year. With increasing experience in the ED, residents improve in performance.[40,41] Residents have been found to see increasing numbers of patients per hour as they progress through their training.[42–47] Increases in productivity by EM residents seem to correlate directly with time spent training in the ED, and not with experience on other rotations.[48] This varying productivity across postgraduate years and resident populations should be a major consideration when designing staffing models in the ED, and may lead to highly variable efficiency depending on which residents are assigned to shifts and the level of attending supervision provided throughout the day. Notably, residents at different stages of their training and in different specialties may preferentially see different kinds of patients, which must also be considered when composing schedules.

Physician shifts in an academic ED also may carry a higher degree of sign-out burden at shift change and variability in resident performance over time. Unlike many community EDs where physicians sign-out a limited number of patients at the end of clinical shifts that are staggered throughout the day, the sign-out burden in an academic setting is typically much greater often times resulting in all ED patients being handed-over from one group of residents to another at shift change.[49] This overall sign-out burden has been observed to contribute to a measurable decrease in resident productivity and requires that faculty critically evaluate the distribution of patients at the time of sign-out to promote resident educational needs, patient safety, and throughput.[50] EM resident productivity has been demonstrated to follow a reliable pattern that shows a significant decrease in patients per hour throughout a single shift, which is preserved across postgraduate years.[47,51] Given the decreased productivity after sign-out and from start to end of shift, operational leaders need to consider innovative approaches, such as staggering resident shifts, to create larger shift overlap and smooth patient flow while protecting the educational value of board rounds, but promoting efficiency and patient safety within an academic setting.[48]

Academic EDs also face unique staffing constraints and opportunities because of Accreditation Council for Graduate Medical Education (ACGME) and Residency Review Committee requirements. The Residency Review Committee requires that faculty members who supervise residents on EM rotations have appropriate qualifications relative to the patient population for which they are providing the supervision. Attendings who are non–American Board of Emergency Medicine/non–American Osteopathic Board of Emergency Medicine certified are only permitted to work in an academic ED if such faculty do not directly supervise residents.[52] The ACGME specifies that academic EDs must maintain sufficient levels of faculty staffing coverage in the ED to ensure "adequate clinical instruction and supervision, and efficient, high quality clinical operations."[53] Acute critical care areas, which are not classified as fast-track or urgent care areas within an academic ED, must have faculty staffing ratio of 4.0 patients per faculty hour or less, which is calculated as described in **Fig. 5**. Further constraining staffing models in academic EDs, the ACGME sets work hour limits for ED residents and requires that residents have a minimum scheduled break time that is equal to the length of the preceding shift. EM residents cannot exceed 72 hours per week of clinical work in the ED. Such requirements reduce flexibility in resident schedules and place additional constraints on schedulers that are not faced in community settings.

Although ED trainees create unique scheduling constraints, trainees also afford academic EDs with opportunities to improve attending productivity and better align staffing to fit the patient-arrival curve. In academic EDs the bulk of patients are seen by residents and then staffed by an attending rather than seen independently by attendings. This pairing of an EM attending with a resident in a one-on-one teaching model allows EM attendings to see significantly more patients per hour than EM physicians alone in the same facility.[54] As a result, staffing models need to take resident and increased attending productivity into account. Although residents each see fewer patients on a shift than an attending there are also a greater number of them staffing the ED. The increased number of providers on a given shift provide academic EDs with the ability to better fit the patient arrival curve and allow for better staffing alignment hour to hour. As such, academic EDs can better adjust to surges throughout the day. Shifting physician coverage hours to match the influx of ED patients can then reduce time-to-provider and improve overall efficiency.[55]

The constant turnover and variability in productivity of physician trainees also requires that academic EDs build processes that are "foolproof" to ensure that process improvement efforts are successfully implemented despite the large number of trainees who provide patient care in the ED only for a single ED rotation. To combat the limited institutional memory that results from the constant turnover of ED trainee physician staff, standardized onboarding processes should exist to train non-EM residents who have rotations in the ED so as to familiarize them with standard operations and reduce variability in physician practice. Residents should be encouraged to use templates to ensure complete documentation and standardize practice. Academic EDs also need to leverage information technology to facilitate

> **(Patient visits per year/faculty hours per day)/365 days per year = Patients per faculty hour[a]**
>
> Example: (70,000 patients per year/55 faculty hours per day)/365 days per year = approximately 3.5 patients per faculty hour

Fig. 5. ACGME-required faculty staffing ratio. [a] Faculty staffing ratios only need to be provided for acute critical care areas, and not for fast track or urgent care areas.

decision support tools, encourage appropriate orders, and reduce wasteful or redundant orders that do not change clinical care and enhance throughput. For example, a variety of academic EDs have used order sets within electronic medical record platforms to eliminate the ordering of amylase by resident physicians. It has been demonstrated that such interventions can greatly reduce the unnecessary ordering of tests that do not add value to patient care.[56] Academic EDs can integrate a variety of decision support tools within their electronic medical records to drive practice patterns and standardize care pathways in alignment with best practices, ensuring that trainees who may not be well versed in EM are guided in their clinical decisions to optimize the quality and safety of patient care and to maintain operational efficiency. Academic EDs can look to partner with other hospital units to design processes in a consistent manner to reduce variability between units and enable trainees to become rapidly familiar with the ED layout and location so as to enhance productivity during ED rotations.[57]

PROMOTING OPERATIONAL RESEARCH WITHIN ACADEMIC EMERGENCY DEPARTMENTS

Academic EDs have the opportunity to improve the quality and efficiency of patient care not only through process improvement efforts, but also by collaborating with faculty scientists to conduct operational research within the ED. Research faculty within academic EDs are often strongly motivated to advance patient care through their research efforts and have experience in measuring care quality and advanced statistical analysis skills that can be repurposed for quality improvement.[58] Promotion criteria also create strong incentives for faculty to invest time and energy in advancing the science of providing high-value care in the ED. Conducting operational research in the ED is challenging because research and operations faculty members commonly work in isolation of one another within the same department. Such divisions often result from differing sources of revenue. Although research groups typically rely heavily on extramural funding, making researchers sensitive to the priorities of granting agencies, operational activities are funded most often through clinical revenue, which rewards immediate clinical and financial outcomes.[59] Leadership within academic EDs must therefore take an innovative approach to promote operationally based scholarly activities if they are to achieve an integrated operational research mission for the department.

ED leadership can take several steps to help promote successful operational research, which include building governance and structure that provides resources and incentives to better align research and operational goals. This includes rewarding ED researchers who involve operational physician leaders in their research programs or work to embed researchers in ED operational initiatives. Researchers should be encouraged to become sensitive to operational metrics when seeking support from operational partners in projects. ED leadership can facilitate an appreciation among operational leadership regarding the potential for research to contribute to developing novel solutions to health care delivery problems. Faculty with operational roles should be encouraged to collaborate with team members from information technology, decision support, or other technologies to improve operational efficiency. Successful academic ED departments promote operational efficiency and redesign of patient care in the ED through operational research and in doing so create an environment that is for optimal academic productivity.

ED operations are a source of quality improvement, resident teaching, and research. ED operations and quality improvement projects, if conducted in a data-driven fashion, can provide a way to introduce residents to operational and research principles. Although the barriers to entry to perform National Institutes of Health–funded research are high and the time commitment is substantial, many ED operations projects have a much shorter cycle time allowing for the involvement of residents in a meaningful way that can fit with their other work demands. Operational projects can reduce many of the difficulties of getting involved with a project because study design and data collection happens in an accelerated fashion that is dependent on patient care imperatives as opposed to relying on resident free time for project progression. In an academic setting, ED operations can serve all three of the missions of an academic center.

SUMMARY

Academic EDs play a critical role in educating future ED physicians, providing cutting-edge emergent care, and conducting research. However, academic EDs and AMCs face enormous challenges because of the decline of governmental funding for research and education and shifting payment models that emphasize efficiency and value.[60] Academic EDs are particularly vulnerable to financial and political changes within government payment programs and declining Centers for Medicare and Medicaid Services reimbursements, because they generally derive a greater proportion of payments from Medicare and Medicaid compared with community EDs. Although academic EDs may have strong reputations within their communities as being affiliated with cutting edge care, they may face lower patient volumes as nonacademic centers develop the capability to evaluate, admit, and perform procedures on patients with a higher degree of medical complexity. Facing such challenges, operational leadership within academic EDs must engage in continuous process improvement efforts to deliver more efficient life-saving care, conduct operational research, and design staffing models that promote education and account for the variability in trainee productivity. In doing so, academic EDs contribute to national efforts to make health care more affordable and become as clinically efficient as possible while supporting their complex tripartite academic mission.[61–63]

DISCLOSURE

The authors have nothing to disclose.

REFERENCES

1. Reznek MA, Scheulen JJ, Harbertson CA, et al. Contributions of academic emergency medicine programs to U.S. health care: summary of the AAAEM-AACEM benchmarking data. Acad Emerg Emerg Med 2018 Apr;25(4):444–52. https://doi.org/10.1111/acem.13337. Epub 2017 Nov 13.
2. Accredited MD Programs in the United States. Liaison Committee on Medical Education. 2017. Available at: http://lcme.org/directory/accredited-u-s-programs/. Accessed October 10, 2019.
3. U.S. Bureau of Labor Statistics. Employment projections, employment by major industry sector, 2006, 2016, and projected 2026 2017. Available at: https://www.bls.gov/emp/tables/employment-by-major-industry-sector.htm. Accessed September 2, 2019.
4. Association of University Technology Managers. Driving the innovation economy. Available at: http://www.autm.net/AUTMMain/media/SurveyReportsPDF/AUTM-FY2016-Infographic-WEB.pdf. Accessed September 30, 2019.

5. Medcalf S. The role of academic health centers in disaster preparedness. Disaster preparedness for seniors. New York: Springer; 2014. p. 261-8.
6. Economic Impact of AAMC Medical Schools and Teaching Hospitals. Available at: https://www.aamc.org/download/488250/data/executive-summary.pdf. Accessed September 12,2019.
7. Beaulieu ND, Joynt KE, Wild R, et al. Concentration of high-cost patients in hospitals and markets. Am J Manag Care 2017;23(4):233-8.
8. Burke L, Khullar D, Orav EJ, et al. Do academic medical centers disproportionately benefit the sickest patients? Health Aff (Millwood) 2018;37(6):864-72.
9. Downey L, Zun L, Burke T, et al. Who pays? How reimbursement impacts the emergency department. J Health Hum Serv Adm 2014;36(4):400-16.
10. Smulowitz P, O'Malley J, Yang X, et al. Increased use of the emergency department after health care reform in Massachusetts. Ann Emerg Med 2014;64: 107-15.
11. Taubman S, Allen H, Wright B, et al. Medicaid increases emergency-department use: evidence from Oregon's health insurance experiment. Science 2014;343: 263-8.
12. Peterson S, Harbertson CA, Scheulen JJ, et al. Trends and characterization of academic emergency department patient visits: a five-year review. Acad Emerg Med 2019;26(4):410-9.
13. Vieth TL, Rhodes KV. The effect of crowding on access and quality in an academic. Am J Emerg Med 2006;24(7):787-94.
14. Klein EY, Levin S, Toerper MF, et al. The effect of Medicaid expansion on utilization in Maryland emergency departments. Ann Emerg Med 2017;17:30784-9.
15. Wiler JL, Welch S, Pine J, et al. Emergency department performance measures updates: proceedings of the 2014 Emergency Medicine Benchmarking Alliance Consensus Summit. Acad Emerg Med 2015;22:542-53.
16. Putera I. Redefining health: implication for value-based healthcare reform. Cureus 2017;9(3):e1067.
17. Mohammed K, Nolan MB, Rajjo T, et al. Creating a Patient-Centered Health Care Delivery System: A Systematic Review of Health Care Quality From the Patient Perspective. Am J Med Qual 2016;31(1):12-21. https://doi.org/10.1177/1062860614545124.
18. Yiadom MY, Baugh CW, Barrett TW, et al. Measuring emergency department acuity. Acad Emerg Med 2018;25:65-75.
19. Kacik A. Available at: https://www.modernhealthcare.com/operations/academic-medical-centers-face-identity-overhaul. Accessed October 15, 2019.
20. Isixsigma. 5 tips for applying Six Sigma from three top hospitals. Available at: https://www.isixsigma.com/industries/healthcare/5-tips-applying-six-sigma-three-top-hospitals/. Accessed September 19, 2019.
21. Burgess N, Radnor Z. Evaluating Lean in healthcare. Int J Health Care Qual Assur 2013;26(3):220-35.
22. Vermeulen MJ, Stukel TA, Guttmann A, et al. Evaluation of an emergency department Lean process improvement program to reduce length of stay. Ann Emerg Med 2014;64:427-38.
23. Kim CS, Spahlinger DA, Kin JM, et al. Lean health care: what can hospitals learn from a world-class automaker? J Hosp Med 2006;1(3):191-9.
24. Aij KH, Simons FE, Widdershoven GA, et al. Experiences of leaders in the implementation of Lean in a teaching hospital-barriers and facilitators in clinical practices: a qualitative study. BMJ Open 2013;3(10):e003605.

25. Antony J, Krishan N, Cullen D, Kumar M. (2012). Lean Six Sigma for higher education institutions (HEIs): Challenges, barriers, success factors, tools/techniques. International Journal of Productivity and Performance Management 2012;61(8): 940–8.

26. Schweikhart SA, Dembe AE. The applicability of Lean and Six Sigma techniques to clinical and translational research. J Investig Med 2009;57:748–55.

27. Stone BK. Four decades of lean: a systematic literature review. International Journal of Lean Six Sigma 2012;3(2):112–32.

28. Mason SE, Nicolay CR, Darzi A. The use of Lean and Six Sigma methodologies in surgery: a systematic review. Surgeon 2015;13:91–100.

29. Roberts J, Fisher T, Trowbridge M, et al. A design thinking framework for healthcare management and innovation. Healthcare 2016;4:11–4.

30. Kolko J. Design thinking comes of age. Harv Bus Rev 2015;93(9):66–71.

31. Furr N, Dyer J. Choose the right innovation method at the right time. Harv Bus Rev 2015. Available at: https://hbr.org/2014/12/choose-the- right-innovation-method-at-the-right-time. Accessed October 11, 2019.

32. Kaplan G, Patterson S. Seeking perfection in healthcare. A case study in adopting Toyota Production System methods. Healthc Exec 2008;23:16–21.

33. Barach P, Philibert I. The July effect: fertile ground for systems improvement. Ann Intern Med 2011;155(5):331–2.

34. Zugar A. Essay: "It's July, the greenest month in hospitals. No need to panic. At New York Times. Science Desk. 2018. Available at: https://www.nytimes.com/1998/07/07/science/essay-it-s-july-the-greenest- month-in-hospitals-no-need-to-panic.html. Accessed October 5, 2019.

35. Deming WE. Quality, productivity, and competitive position. Cambridge (MA): MIT Press; 1982.

36. DiBiase LM, Weber DJ, Sickbert-Bennett EE, et al. July effect: impact of the academic year-end changeover on the incidence of healthcare-associated infections. Infect Control Hosp Epidemiol 2014;35(03):321–2.

37. Phillips DP, Barker GE. A July spike in fatal medication errors: a possible effect of new medical residents. J Gen Intern Med 2010;25(8):774–9.

38. O'Halloran PL. Performance pay and employee turnover. J Econ Stud 2012;39(6): 653–74.

39. Chopra S, Kondapalli M. Applying lean principles to mitigate the "July Effect": addressing challenges associated with cohort turnover in teaching hospitals. J Technol Manag;2015, Appl Eng 34(2).

40. Riguzzi C, Hern HG, Vahidnia F, et al. The July effect: is emergency department length of stay greater at the beginning of the hospital academic year? West J Emerg Med 2014;15(1):88.

41. Bahl A, Catherine Cooley Hixson C. July phenomenon impacts efficiency of emergency care. West J Emerg Med 2019;20(1):157–62.

42. Dowd MD, Tarantino C, Barnett TM, et al. Resident efficacy in a pediatric emergency department. Acad Emerg Med 2005;12(12):1240–4.

43. Thibodeau LG, Geary SP, Werter C. An evaluation of resident work profiles, attending-resident teaching interactions, and the effect of variations in emergency department volume on each. Acad Emerg Med 2010;17(Suppl 2):S62–6.

44. Chan L, Kass LE. Impact of medical student preceptorship on ED patient throughput time. Am J Emerg Med 1999;17:41–3.

45. McGarry J, Krall S, McLaughlin T. Impact of resident physicians on emergency department throughput. West J Emerg Med 2010;11(4):333–5.

46. Schafer AI. The fault lines of academic medicine. Perspect Biol Med 2002;45(3): 416–25.

47. Henning D, McGillicuddy D, Sanchez LD. Evaluating the effect of emergency residency training on productivity in the emergency department. J Emerg Med 2013; 45(3):414–8.

48. Joseph JW, Chiu DT, Wong ML, et al. Experience within the emergency department and improved productivity for first year residents in emergency medicine and other specialties. West J Emerg Med 2018;19(1):128–33.

49. Joseph JW, Stenson BA, Wong ML, et al. The effect of signed out emergency department patients on resident productivity. J Emerg Med 2018;55(2):244–51.

50. Joseph JW, Novack V, Wong ML, et al. Do slow and steady residents win the race? Modeling the effects of peak and overall resident productivity in the emergency department. J Emerg Med 2017;53(2):252–9.

51. Jeanmonod R, Brook C, Winther M, et al. Resident productivity as a function of emergency department volume, shift time of day, and cumulative time in the emergency department. Am J Emerg Med 2009;27(3):313–9.

52. ACGME common program requirements (residency). Available at: https://acgme. org/Portals/0/PFAssets/ProgramRequirements/CPRResidency2019.pdf. Accessed September 15, 2019.

53. ACGME program requirements for graduate medical education in emergency medicine. Available at: https://www.acgme.org/Portals/0/PFAssets/ ProgramRequirements/110_EmergencyMedicine_2019.pdf?ver=2019-06-25- 082649-063. Accessed September 15, 2019.

54. Bhat R, DUbin J, Maloy K. Impact of learners on emergency medicine attending physician productivity. West J Emerg Med 2014;15(1):41–4.

55. Green LV, Soares J, Giglio JF, et al. Using queueing theory to increase the effectiveness of emergency department provider staffing. Acad Emerg Med 2006; 13(1):61–8.

56. Volz KA, McGillicuddy DC, Horowitz GL, et al. Creatine kinase-MB does not add additional benefit to a negative troponin in the evaluation of chest pain. Am J Emerg Med 2012;30(1):188–90.

57. Sadler BL, DuBose J, Craig Z. The business case for building better hospitals through evidence-based design. HERD 2008;1(3):22–39.

58. Yeh H-C, Bertram A, Brancati FL, et al. Perceptions of division directors in general internal medicine about the importance of and support for scholarly work done by clinician-educators. Acad Med 2015;90(2):203–8.

59. Mann D, Hess R. Academic medical center R&D: a call for creating an operational research infrastructure within the academic medical center. Clin Transl Sci 2015;8(6):871–2.

60. Nuckols T, Weingarten S, Priselac T. What value-based payment means for academic medical centers. 2019. Available at:https://catalyst.nejm.org/doi/full/10. 1056/CAT.19.0656. Accessed September 15, 2019.

61. Adams JF, Biros MH. The elusive nature of quality. Acad Emerg Med 2002;9: 1067–70.

62. Beach C, Leon H, Adams J, et al. Clinical operations in academic emergency medicine. Acad Emerg Med 2003;10(7):806–7.

63. Bucci S, de Belvis AG, Marventano S, et al. Emergency department crowding and hospital bed shortage: is Lean a smart answer? A systematic review. Eur Rev Med Pharmacol Sci 2016;20(20):4209–19.

Strategies for Provider Well-Being in the Emergency Department

Matthew L. Wong, MD, MPH[a],*, Arlene S. Chung, MD, MACM[b]

KEYWORDS

- Wellness • Emergency medicine • Stress • Burnout

KEY POINTS

- Circadian disruption is a significant cause of decreased performance and long-term burnout among emergency physicians. Administrators should help to schedule shifts in a way that minimizes short turn-around times after night shifts and should consider breaking up overnight shifts into smaller portions that allow for some sleep.
- Emergency physicians tend to see fewer patients late in their shifts, which parallels decreasing performance and productivity with fatigue seen in other professions with a heavy cognitive load. Work strategies that promote decreasing responsibility over the course of a shift, such as seeing less-acute patients later on, may help to mitigate this effect.
- Workplace violence remains a serious, underappreciated issue faced by emergency physicians and nurses. Administrators need to advocate for proactive measures to ensure the safety of clinical staff.
- Unexpected family crises and the ever-present risk of malpractice are serious stressors that can contribute to burnout and other long-lasting consequences for emergency physicians. Administrators should make plans to help support colleagues who face these stressors rather than expecting them to push through on their own.

INTRODUCTION: PROMOTING WELLNESS

Over the past decade, the concept of "burnout," a syndrome characterized by stress, fatigue, depersonalization, and cynicism, has gone from a niche term discussed primarily in psychological research to an open topic of discussion among emergency physicians (EPs) and has found its way into residency curricula and yearly talks at major emergency medicine conferences. The term continues to gain traction in the broader medical and surgical community, as an issue in professional practice, and

[a] Department of Emergency Medicine, Beth Israel Deaconess Medical Center, One Deaconess Road, Boston, MA 02215, USA; [b] Department of Emergency Medicine, Maimonides Medical Center, Brooklyn, NY, USA
* Corresponding author.
E-mail address: MLWong@bidmc.harvard.edu

Emerg Med Clin N Am 38 (2020) 729–738
https://doi.org/10.1016/j.emc.2020.03.005
0733-8627/20/© 2020 Elsevier Inc. All rights reserved.

increasingly, as a longitudinal challenge of medical education. The American College of Emergency Physicians (ACEP) published an extensive guide on well-being in emergency medicine a few years ago, and the National Academy of Medicine has written extensively on the subject as well.[1,2]

Much of the current discourse on wellness and burnout within emergency medicine has been on developing frameworks to understand what it means to be "well" and have a career in medicine, quantifying the severity of the problems, and developing a research agenda to better understand the threats that burnout poses to patients and to EPs' longevity.[3] Although what it means to be "well" is distinctly personal, the root causes of burnout are systemic problems, imposed by the mismatch between EPs' substantial professional responsibilities and the relatively insubstantial support they receive from hospitals and the larger health care system.[4]

Among the most corrosive forces contributing to burnout are those of "moral injury," feelings of distress resulting from physicians being compelled to provide care that they think is substandard. The reality of working in a crowded emergency department (ED) provides many such opportunities, an EP may think that she cannot provide her patients with her full attention while managing a boarding intensive care unit patient, whereas hospital management tells her that the appropriate response to crowding is simply to work faster. Not surprisingly, several prominent writers have highlighted that many organizations within modern health care thrive by exploiting the inherent good nature of physicians.[5,6]

Unfortunately, despite the depth of the problem of burnout, solutions to address root causes and mitigate its negative effects are scant.[7] In a recent review of wellness interventions, most interventions attempting to address burnout involved duty-hour restrictions for trainees (with little relevance to attending physicians in practice), and programs to promote mindfulness, stress management, improving peer-to-peer support, and professional coaching for individuals.[7,8]

What should a practicing EP (or a local leader of a department of EPs) do? Some sources of stress and insult are larger than any particular department or hospital, such as payer reimbursement or the local malpractice environment. However, the literature shows that the issues that are most important to us are surprisingly local and may fall within the control of administrators. A disproportionate amount of burnout (and enjoyment from work) comes down to the day-to-day working environment. With this principle in mind, the authors highlight the following areas where local physician-leaders can really make a difference in physician well-being.

CIRCADIAN RHYTHM AND SHIFT WORK

Shift work is both a draw to the specialty of emergency medicine and a source of distress. The mission to take care of patients regardless of circumstance includes the provision that they can receive quality care at any time, including evenings, overnights, weekends, and holidays. Working from 9 in the morning to 5 o'clock at night from Monday to Friday may represent the quintessential workday for other professionals, but most of the hours of a week fall outside that window, and so EPs work predominantly outside those hours. In particular, working overnight is major source of stress for physicians. Individuals report that night shifts negatively affect their health, contribute to fatigue and poor-quality sleep, and are a contributing factor as to when individual EPs retire from the job.[9] Because this is an important issue for wellness, and because the shift schedule is mostly under local control, administrators involved in ED operations need to understand scheduling shifts cannot simply be a matter of maximizing efficiency: wellness must be a primary endpoint of scheduling.

For many people shift work causes a pathologic form of sleep. The American Academy of Sleep Medicine recognizes "shift-work disorder" as a disease, and the World Health Organization recognizes nighttime work as a probable carcinogen.[10,11] In the Nurses' Health Study (a very large prospective cohort of registered nurses commonly used in epidemiology), researchers found that rotating night shift work increased the risk of all-cause mortality.[12]

Specifically with an eye toward well-being, the ACEP recommends forward circadian rhythm scheduling (scheduling progressively later shifts), limiting shift length, limiting long stretches of shifts, prioritizing the health and adequately compensating overnight workers, and providing a safe space to sleep after night shifts.[13] Although many departments have tailored the hours of the shifts in their department to fit their local needs, there have been no significant trials examining the design of shift structures to promote wellness or career longevity. In a study of emergency medicine residents, there was substantial variability in terms of their scheduling preferences.[14] Shorter shifts come at the cost of an increased number of shifts, whereas longer shifts may come at the cost of fatigue. Each department needs to consider multiple factors when designing shift schedules and balancing clinical work and time off. However, in a large longitudinal study of Diplomates of the American Board of Emergency Medicine, physical fatigue, the number of night shifts, and the length of shifts were the strongest predictors of burnout.[15]

To reduce the fatigue of working an overnight shift, some departments have adopted "casino shifts" in lieu of traditional shifts.[16] Traditional overnight shifts start in the evening hours and last until the early morning (eg, 2200 hours or 2300 hours until 0700 hours, or 1900 hours until 0700 hours). This traditional overnight shift is very disruptive to circadian rhythm cycles because the person working overnight is completely misaligned from normal sleep cycles. The casino shift essentially splits the overnight into 2 shorter shifts. Instead of a single 2200 hour to 0700 hour shift, 1 doctor would work from 2200 hours to 0400 hours, and then a second doctor would work from 0400 hours until 1000 hours. This arrangement would allow both doctors to sleep at least some part of the time while it was dark outside. When implemented at 1 hospital, the results were impressive (although only published in abstract form): 87% of the EPs preferred casino shift scheduling, as did 63% of their families, and the doctors slept more after their shift (6 vs 4.5 hours), and the perceived recovery time was less (1.2 vs 2.1 days).[17]

Aside from the issues of fatigue and inconvenience when optimizing shift scheduling, data suggest that the marginal productivity of physicians changes significantly while working. With each passing hour on shift, physician productivity declines significantly.[18,19] Emergency medicine is mentally demanding, and during the midpoint of a shift, an EP's new patient-per-hour productivity is roughly half that compared with the beginning of the shift and continues to drop in each subsequent hour.[19]

This decrease in productivity may represent a cognitive defense mechanism to limit the exposure of work and limit mental burden, but may also reflect the fact that although EPs are expected to see new patients at a consistent rate, patient workups may stretch over the course of many hours, necessitating an increasing degree of physician multitasking as the shift continues. The ability to make decisions decreases as a shift wears on.[20] An example of this can be found in the prescribing pattern for antibiotics by primary care physicians for acute respiratory tract infections throughout the day. Because it is cognitively easier to prescribe an antibiotic for what is likely a viral infection (instead of taking the risk of upsetting the patient, or taking take time to explain the medical decision making), physicians are more likely to prescribe antibiotics for acute respiratory infection later in the day than in the beginning of the day.[21] This same phenomena has recently been demonstrated in EPs' willingness to admit patients during a shift. Compared with earlier in the shift, EPs are more likely to admit a patient later on in their shift than earlier, perhaps because it is cognitively easier to do so than to discharge the patient and risk an adverse event.[22]

This phenomenon parallels a famous study in psychology that examined the determinants of receiving a favorable decision for parole. For a judge, the decision to grant a prisoner parole is associated with more risk and mental work than maintaining the prisoner's current position in jail. Independent of other factors, the decision to grant a prisoner parole (vs keep them in custody or defer the decision to a later date) was associated with the time of day and the judge's proximity to a break. Prisoners who had their case reviewed early in the day and immediately after a break had the best chance of getting parole.[23] The title of this article was "Extraneous factors in judicial decisions." It is time to consider that extraneous factors contribute to medical decision making, and what can be done to limit these negative influences should be considered.

VIOLENCE IN THE EMERGENCY DEPARTMENT

Gun violence is a persistent and disquieting issue that continues to grow, despite increased awareness and efforts to limit firearm access. Schools and communities have shared the grief following tragedies such as Columbine and Sandy Hook. Hospital personnel not only care for the victims from these events but also have been the targets of violence as well. On January 20, 2015, a man of unremarkable height, weight, and appearance walked into Brigham and Women's Hospital in Boston, Massachusetts and asked to see Dr Michael J. Davidson.[24] The man opened fire when the cardiovascular surgeon stepped into an examination room to speak with him, and both men died.

The ED and psychiatric wards are places where health care providers are often verbally or physically injured while at work.[25] The ACEP as well as the Emergency Nurses Association has studied the issue, and in a recent poll of more than 35,000 EPs nationwide, nearly half of the respondents had been physically assaulted.[26] Ninety-six percent of all women and 80% of all men EPs reported that they had been the victim of inappropriate comments or unwanted advances toward them. Verbal threats and physical assault are also common in residents.[27]

The negative effects of these interactions contribute to burnout, depression, and posttraumatic stress in physicians.[28,29] Most hospitals do not have metal detectors at their entrances. Long wait times, high-stress situations, and short fuses compound the anxiety and frustration felt by both patients and visitors, making EDs particularly susceptible to workplace violence. Nurses suffer significantly more verbal and physical assault compared with physicians, sometimes more than twice as frequently in some studies, although the rates for physicians are also high.[30,31] Gates and colleagues[31] found that 51% of physicians reported at least 1 episode of physical violence against them within that past 12 months. Given the known tendency for underreporting of events, individuals rationalizing that this is just "part of the job" of working in an ED, the actual incidence of workplace violence is likely even higher. Another study of 6 different EDs found that 20% of verbal threats to any staff member resulted in physical injury.[30]

According to the study by Gates and colleagues,[31] not surprisingly, alcohol intoxication, drug use, and psychiatric illness have been cited as the most frequent risk factors for perpetrators of abuse against health care workers. Most assaults occur overnight and increase with increasing wait times. As an additional concern, 25% of violent episodes were related to the ease of ability to bring weapons into the ED.

Not only does workplace violence cause obvious physical distress to those involved but also it can create an environment in which health care workers feel unsafe. Of the different types of staff in the ED, patient representatives have the highest percentage of workers (60%) who report feeling unsafe.[31] In general terms, there is an inverse relationship between feelings of safety, all types of violence, and job satisfaction. Acute stress symptoms are most prevalent in staff that reports the greatest frequency of verbal and physical threats and assaults.[30]

Prevention strategies to address workplace violence include specific training of medical staff to recognize signs of violence, modification of the actual physical structure of the ED, and policy development.[30] Surveyed health care workers reported that they would like to see an increased police presence and more physical barriers, such as metal detectors.[31]

FAMILY AND MEDICAL LEAVE

Over half of the US population is female; women comprise more than half of medical student matriculants, and 38% of all emergency medicine residents are women.[32,33] Young physicians have drastically different attitudes about having children and a career in medicine compared with prior generations. In 1980, only 13% of female graduate medical education trainees became pregnant during their training, but that number has nearly tripled to 35% nationally, and in some institutions and in some specific residencies that number is even higher.[34] Even among men, 93% of millennial-generation new fathers think that paternity leave is important, compared with 77% of baby boomers.[35]

Despite the secular change in opinion, the workplace is a source of stress and discrimination for many new parents, and particularly for new mothers. In a recent survey, 36% of all female physicians experienced discrimination based on pregnancy, maternity leave, or breast feeding.[36] The ACEP recommends that every ED, physician group, and residency should have a policy about family leave, and furthermore, that it guarantees at least 12 weeks' paid time off for new mothers, and 4 weeks of paid time off for other parents.[37]

The United States is the rare exception to the global consensus that parental leave is not guaranteed for everyone.[38] The US federal Family and Medical Leave Act does not apply to employees of a company less than 50 individuals (which would excludes those employed by a small physician group), only if they have worked in their place of employment for a year and for 1250 hours (which would exclude new graduates and part-time employees), and does not apply to individuals paid through an independent contractor mechanism (as many EPs are).[39]

There are no randomized controlled trials regarding the effects of parental leave on the productivity or well-being of EPs. However, there does not necessarily have to be any for us to act. This topic is important for many EPs and is an easy way for EPs to take care of each other and improve their collective well-being.

The most common concerns that prevent the expansion of parental leave involve finances and work productivity. Specifically, this includes issues related to how the physician going to be compensated while on leave, where that money is going to come from, and who is going to cover the shifts for the time that they are gone. This problem is complex and is particularly difficult because each group or organization pays physicians through different accounting strategies, and some EPs work under an independent contractor model. Some known practices include using short-term disability insurance to finance part of the leave, using saved department coffers, and rebalancing an individual's shift allotments to average out a full-time complement but over a longer period of time.

Besides birth mothers, other partners in relationships may also benefit directly from parental leave.[38] Moreover, mandating them to take leave may be important. In the example of a heterosexual relationship, labor practices that provide women parental leave but do not provide for parental leave might exacerbate long-standing gender inequities and workplace sexism.[40] If the workplace permits women to take maternity leave but it does not provide adequate time for men to take care of newborns, then an unequal amount of childcare burden is shifted to women, which is the opposite effect than intended. To combat the problem of structured gender inequity, several Scandinavian countries have experimented with the concept of mandatory paternity leave with so-called father's quota, although the concept has not gained traction in the United States yet.

Even upon returning to the workplace, many women face discrimination and barriers to pumping breast milk.[36] The American Academy of Pediatrics recommends that newborns exclusively receive breast milk for 6 months, and they should continue to receive breast milk until at least they are 1 year old.[41] EDs need to be supportive of new mothers during this time and should be accommodating. The ACEP supports nursing mothers and recommends a private area for women to express milk that is not the bathroom and that is in proximity to the department.[42]

In closing, a robust parental leave policy, and associated cultural change that supports parents on returning to work, is paramount to combating burnout and making physicians feel valued as individuals. With the recent national emphasis on wellness and job satisfaction, it would be prudent for departments to come up with a coherent strategy and invest time and resources into this issue.

LITIGATION STRESS

A 2016 study conducted by the American Medical Association found that more than 52% of US EPs reported having been sued at least once and more than 26% report being sued 2 or more times.[43] These rates were much higher than the mean across all specialties, which were 34% and 17%, respectively. Residents can be sued too. A study in the *Journal of the American Medical Association* estimated that residents have been named in approximately 22% of lawsuits.[44] In most cases, they are named as codefendants with the attending physician on the case and may be held to the same standards of care. Although the attending is usually determined to be ultimately responsible for the care of the patient, malpractice lawsuits may become part of the resident's permanent professional record should the claim result in payment.[45]

Cognitive, Behavioral, and Affective Consequences of Litigation Stress

The looming specter of malpractice casts a long shadow, including affecting physicians who have not been served. Many physicians admit to practicing defensive medicine, referring to the practice of performing a diagnostic test or treatment that primarily serves the function of protecting the physician against possible future litigation, rather than the best interests of the patient's health. EPs in particular practice in an information-poor, high-risk, technology-rich environment that lends itself to defensive decision making. This environment inevitably leads to increased costs and a greater rate of false-positive findings that may adversely affect patients. Unfortunately, this culture has become so engrained, that even with tort reform, physicians continue to practice defensively.[46]

Merely the threat of being sued may contribute to decreased career longevity. One study found that EPs cited malpractice and litigation stress as one of the top 3 reasons for burnout and a desire to leave the field.[47] Furthermore, as this study and many others have found, physicians who report high levels of burnout are also more likely to retire early.

There are real physical, mental, and emotional costs to being sued as a physician. Medical malpractice stress syndrome (MMSS) shares many features of posttraumatic stress disorder.[48,49] Victims suffer psychological distress, often manifesting as anxiety and depression, and may also experience physical symptoms, such as the development of a new physical illness or exacerbation of a preexisting one, such as diabetes or hypertension. Physicians with MMSS report feelings of isolation, negative self-image, irritability, and difficulty concentrating. They may experience insomnia, fatigue, or hyperexcitability. They may be prone to compulsively overordering tests on patients and consider changing careers. Physicians with MMSS may resort to self-medication with alcohol or recreational drugs and in extreme cases may contemplate, or complete, suicide. Finally, although MMSS is not ubiquitous among physicians who have been sued, almost all will experience at least some form of depression, anger, shame, or feelings of isolation, which is independent of whether or not any negligence, real or imagined by the physician involved, actually occurred.

Strategies for Mitigating Litigation Stress

Demystification of the legal process can be effective in reducing anxiety. Representatives from the hospital risk-management department should be readily available to answer questions from defendants. Resources such as published books and journal articles can also be good sources of information about the litigation process.

Many risk-management groups offer confidential peer-counseling networks. Often conducted over the telephone, within the confidential peer-counseling networks, physicians can anonymously contact another physician who has also been sued in the past. This confidential peer-counseling network not only provides a means of sharing emotions with a truly empathic individual but it also serves as another means of learning more about the litigation process and what to expect.

It can be useful to seek treatment from a licensed mental health professional and most certainly for thoughts of persistent depression, guilt, hopelessness, thoughts of self-harm, and any of the symptoms consistent with MMSS. The confidential peer-counseling network can provide a source of emotional support, safe space for brainstorming effective coping strategies, and prescribe medications if necessary.

SUMMARY

There are many aspects that contribute to provider well-being in the ED, and it is paramount for ED leaders to remain cognizant of the fact that their decisions can have significant effects on physician wellness. Although the concept of "wellness" may seem vague, theoretical, or intangible at times, many of the most important contributing factors are well within the control of ED leadership, and developing robust and supportive structures and culture can make a big difference in the lives of individual physicians.

DISCLOSURE

The authors have nothing to disclose.

REFERENCES

1. ACEP. Being well in emergency medicine: ACEP's guide to investing in yourself. 2017. Available at: https://www.acep.org/globalassets/sites/acep/media/wellness/acepwellnessguide.pdf. Accessed November 1, 2019.
2. Dyrbye LN, Shanafelt TD, Sinsky CA, et al. Burnout among health care professionals: a call to explore and address this underrecognized threat to safe. Washington, DC: High-Quality Care; 2017. https://doi.org/10.31478/201707b.
3. Chung AS, Wong ML, Sanchez LD, et al. Research priorities for physician wellness in academic emergency medicine: consensus from the Society for Academic Emergency Medicine Wellness Committee. AEM Educ Train 2018;1–8. https://doi.org/10.1002/aet2.10211.
4. Shanafelt TD, Mungo M, Schmitgen J, et al. Longitudinal study evaluating the association. Mayo Clin Proc 2016;91:422–31.
5. Talbot S, Dean W. Physicians aren't 'burning out.' They're suffering from moral injury. STAT News 2018. Available at: https://www.statnews.com/2018/07/26/physicians-not-burning-out-they-are-suffering-moral-injury/. Accessed September 1, 2019.
6. Ofri D. The business of health care depends on exploiting doctors and nurses. New York Times 2019. Available at: https://nyti.ms/31ma6Qz.
7. West CP, Dyrbye LN, Rabatin JT, et al. Intervention to promote physician well-being, job satisfaction, and professionalism. JAMA Intern Med 2014;174(4):527.
8. Dyrbye LN, Shanafelt TD, Gill PR, et al. Effect of a professional coaching intervention on the well-being and distress of physicians: a pilot randomized clinical trial. JAMA Intern Med 2019. https://doi.org/10.1001/jamainternmed.2019.2425.
9. Smith-Coggins R, Broderick KB, Marco CA. Night shifts in emergency medicine: the American Board of Emergency Medicine Longitudinal Study of Emergency Physicians. J Emerg Med 2014;47(3):372–8.
10. Sack RL, Auckley D, Auger RR, et al. Circadian rhythm sleep disorders: part I, basic principles, shift work and jet lag disorders. Sleep 2007;30(11):1460–83.
11. Straif K, Baan R, Grosse Y, et al. Carcinogenicity of shift-work, painting, and fire-fighting. Lancet Oncol 2007;8(12):1065–6.
12. Gu F, Han J, Laden F, et al. Total and cause-specific mortality of U.S. nurses working rotating night shifts. Am J Prev Med 2015;48(3):241–52.
13. ACEP. Emergency physician shift work. Ann Emerg Med 2017;70. https://doi.org/10.1016/j.annemergmed.2017.08.028.
14. Rischall ML, Chung AS, Tabatabai R, et al. Emergency medicine resident shift work preferences: a comparison of resident scheduling preferences and recommended schedule design for shift workers. AEM Educ Train 2018;2(3):229–35.
15. Cydulka RK, Korte R. Career satisfaction in emergency medicine: the ABEM Longitudinal Study of Emergency Physicians. Ann Emerg Med 2008;51(6):714–22.e1.
16. Ross S, Liu EL, Rose C, et al. Strategies to enhance wellness in emergency medicine residency training programs. Ann Emerg Med 2017;70(6):891–7.
17. Croskerry P, Sinclair D. Casino shift-scheduling in the emergency department: a strategy for abolishing the night-shift? Emerg Med J 2002;19(Suppl 1):A9. Available at: http://emj.bmj.com/content/suppl/2002/08/28/19.4.DC2/abs34to75.pdf.
18. Joseph JW, Davis S, Wilker EH, et al. Modelling attending physician productivity in the emergency department: a multicentre study. Emerg Med J 2018. https://doi.org/10.1136/emermed-2017-207194. emermed-2017-207194.

19. Joseph JW, Henning DJ, Strouse CS, et al. Modeling hourly resident productivity in the emergency department. Ann Emerg Med 2017;70(2):185–90.e6.
20. Muraven M, Baumeister RF. Self-regulation and depletion of limited resources: does self-control resemble a muscle? Psychol Bull 2000;126(2):247–59.
21. Linder JA, Doctor JN, Friedberg MW, et al. Time of day and the decision to prescribe antibiotics. JAMA Intern Med 2014;174(12):2029–31.
22. Tyler PD, Fossa A, Joseph JW, et al. Later emergency provider shift hour is associated with increased risk of admission: a retrospective cohort study. BMJ Qual Saf 2019. https://doi.org/10.1136/bmjqs-2019-009546 [pii:bmjqs-2019-009546].
23. Danziger S, Levav J, Avnaim-Pesso L. Extraneous factors in judicial decisions. Proc Natl Acad Sci U S A 2011;108(17):6889–92.
24. Freyer FJ, Kowalczyk L, Murphy S. Surgeon slain, gunman found dead in day of crisis at Brigham. Boston, MA: Boston Globe; 2015.
25. Phillips JP. Workplace violence against health care workers in the United States. N Engl J Med 2016;374(17):1661–9.
26. American College of Emergency Physicians. Emergency department violence poll research results. 2018. Available at: https://www.emergencyphysicians.org/globalassets/files/pdfs/2018acep-emergency-department-violence-pollresults-2.pdf. Accessed November 1, 2019.
27. Schnapp BH, Slovis BH, Shah AD, et al. Workplace violence and harassment against emergency medicine residents. West J Emerg Med 2016;17(5):567–73.
28. Sui G, Liu G, Jia L, et al. Associations of workplace violence and psychological capital with depressive symptoms and burn-out among doctors in Liaoning, China: a cross-sectional study. BMJ Open 2019;9(5):e024186.
29. Zafar W, Khan UR, Siddiqui SA, et al. Workplace violence and self-reported psychological health: coping with post-traumatic stress, mental distress, and burnout among physicians working in the emergency departments compared to other specialties in Pakistan. J Emerg Med 2016;50(1):167–77.e1.
30. Kowalenko T, Cunningham R, Sachs CJ, et al. Workplace violence in emergency medicine: current knowledge and future directions. J Emerg Med 2012;43(3): 523–31.
31. Gates DM, Ross CS, McQueen L. Violence against emergency department workers. J Emerg Med 2006;31(3):331–7.
32. American Association of Medical. 2018 fall applicant and matriculant data tables 2018. Available at: https://www.aamc.org/system/files/d/1/92-applicant_and_matriculant_data_tables.pdf. Accessed October 1, 2019.
33. Parker RB, Stack SJ, Schneider SM, et al. Why diversity and inclusion are critical to the American College of Emergency Physicians' future success. Ann Emerg Med 2017;69(6):714–7.
34. Blair JE, Mayer AP, Caubet SL, et al. Pregnancy and parental leave during graduate medical education. Acad Med 2016;91(7):972–8.
35. Harrington B, Van Deusen F, Eddy S, et al. The new dad: take your leave. Perspectives on paternity leave from fathers, leading organizations, and global policies. 2018. Available at: http://www.thenewdad.org/yahoo_site_admin/assets/docs/BCCWF_The_New_Dad_2014_FINAL.157170735.pdf. Accessed November 1, 2019.
36. Adesoye T, Mangurian C, Choo EK, et al. Perceived discrimination experienced by physician mothers and desired workplace changes. JAMA Intern Med 2017; 177(7):1033.
37. American College of Emergency Physicians. Family and medical leave. Ann Emerg Med 2019;74(5):e103.

38. International Labour Organization. Maternity and paternity at work: law and practice across the world. 2014. Available at: https://www.ilo.org/global/publications/ilo-bookstore/order-online/books/WCMS_242615/lang–en/index.htm.

39. Family and Medical Leave Act of 1993. Available at: https://www.dol.gov/agencies/whd/laws-and-regulations/laws/fmla.

40. Rønsen M, Kitterød RH. Gender-equalizing family policies and mothers' entry into paid work: recent evidence from Norway. Fem Econ 2015;21(1):59–89.

41. American Academy of Pediatrics. Breastfeeding and the use of human milk. Pediatrics 2012;129(3):e827–41.

42. American College of Emergency Physicians. Support for nursing mothers. Ann Emerg Med 2015;65(1):129.

43. American Medical Association. Medical liability claim frequency among U.S. physicians. 2017. Available at: https://www.ama-assn.org/sites/ama-assn.org/files/corp/media-browser/public/government/advocacy/policy-research-perspective-medical-liability-claim-frequency.pdf.

44. Kachalia A, Studdert DM. Professional liability issues in graduate medical education. JAMA 2004;292(9):1051–6.

45. Bailey RA. Resident liability in medical malpractice. Ann Emerg Med 2013;61(1):114–7.

46. Levin ML. The effect of malpractice reform on emergency department care. N Engl J Med 2015;372(2):191.

47. Doan-Wiggins L, Zun L, Cooper MA, et al. Practice satisfaction, occupational stress, and attrition of emergency physicians. Wellness Task Force, Illinois College of Emergency Physicians. Acad Emerg Med 1995;2(6):556–63. https://doi.org/10.1111/j.1553-2712.1995.tb03261.x.

48. Kelly JD. Malpractice stress. Orthopedics 2008;31(10).

49. Medical malpractice stress syndrome. In: Sanbar S, Firestone M, Wecht C, et al, editors. The medical malpractice survival handbook. Elsevier; 2007. p. 9–15. https://doi.org/10.1016/B978-0-323-04438-7.X5001-3. Available at: https://www.google.com/books/edition/The_Medical_Malpractice_Survival_Handboo/1XijBQAAQBAJ?hl=en&gbpv=0.

Moving?

Make sure your subscription moves with you!

To notify us of your new address, find your **Clinics Account Number** (located on your mailing label above your name), and contact customer service at:

Email: journalscustomerservice-usa@elsevier.com

800-654-2452 (subscribers in the U.S. & Canada)
314-447-8871 (subscribers outside of the U.S. & Canada)

Fax number: 314-447-8029

Elsevier Health Sciences Division
Subscription Customer Service
3251 Riverport Lane
Maryland Heights, MO 63043

*To ensure uninterrupted delivery of your subscription, please notify us at least 4 weeks in advance of move.

Printed and bound by CPI Group (UK) Ltd, Croydon, CR0 4YY

03/10/2024

01040481-0018